A Guide to Change Your Life
with Practical Techniques
for Physical and Mental Well-being

The History, Cultivation &
Practice of Qigong

QIGONG REVOLUTION

Author & Editor: Byung Joo Choi
Translator: Sang P. Han
Illustrator: Hee Jung Han
Published by Golden Rishi Academy USA

Golden Rishi Qigong & Tai Chi
For more information, contact: info@goldenrishi.com
Website: Goldenrishi.com

Golden Rishi
QIGONG REVOLUTION

Breathing and meditation to master the body and mind

Ma-ae stone monument to Korean sage Kim Gagi, discovered in Jaogou, Ziwugu of Sungseosng, China.

Contents

Contents 5
Foreword 7
Acknowledgements 13
Preface 14
Part I. Golden Rishi Qigong Principles and History
   Chapter I. What is Qigong? 1
      A. The Origin of Qigong 1
      B. Exploring the Structure of Qigong 4
         1. What is Innate Nature? 5
         2. What is Cultivation of Life? (命) 12
         3. Essence, Energy, Spirit and Ethereal & Corporeal Soul ... 16
   Chapter II. The History and Origin of Qigong 23
      A. The History of Qigong 24
      B. The Roots of Qigong 30
      C. Prospects for the Future 36
      D. History of Seon Do 41
         1. History of Seon Do in China 41
         2. History of Seon Do in Korea 47
   Chapter III. Principles of Qigong 62
      A. Refining Essence and Transforming Qi 64
      B. Refining Qi and Transforming Spirit 77
      C. Cultivating the Spirit and Returning to Emptiness 91
      D. Cultivating Emptiness and Harmonizing with the Dao 95
   Chapter IV. Seon Do: Way of Immortals 100
      A. What is Seon Do? Why Should Humans Practice Seon Do? ... 101
      B. Overview of Sojucheon and Kundalini 104
      C. About the Energy Centers 110
         1. Coccygeal Plexus (Seminal Vesicle-Males/Womb-Females) ... 110
         2. Sacral Plexus (Spermatic Cord, Ovaries) 114

3. Solar Plexus (Adrenal Glands) 115
　　　4. Thoracic Plexus (Thymus) 116
　　　5. Throat Plexus (Thyroid) 120
　　　6. Hypothalamus (Pineal Gland) 121
　　　7. The Entire Cerebrum (大腦) 123
　　D. Sojucheon / Kundalini 127
　　E. Purpose of the Practice 133
Chapter V. Principles of the Internal Organs 144
　　A. The Nature of the Internal Organs 145
　　　1. The five organs (五臟) 152
　　　2. The six bowels (六腑) 161
　　B. The Non-organ System (奇恒之腑) 167
　　　1. Brain (腦) 167
　　　2. Marrow (髓) 168
　　　3. Bones (骨) 169
　　　4. Vessels (脈) 169
　　C. Harmonizing the Internal Organs (臟腑) 170
　　D. Internal Organs (臟腑) and the Nine Outlets (九竅) 170
　　　1. The Ears (耳) 171
　　　2. The Eyes (目) 172
　　　3. The Nose (鼻) 173
　　　4. The Mouth (口) 174
　　　5. The Tongue (舌) 174
　　　6. The Anterior Perineum (前陰) 175
　　　7. The Posterior Perineum (後陰) 175

Part II. Golden Rishi Qigong Training

Chapter VI. Course of Practice 179
Chapter VII. Seated Meditation 187
　　A. Sitting Posture 187
　　　1. Natural Sitting Posture 188
　　　2. Half Lotus Sitting Posture 189
　　　3. Golden Rishi Sitting Posture 189
　　　4. Lotus Sitting Posture 190
　　B. Breathing Methods 193
Chapter VIII. Breathing Techniques 205

  A. Breathing Method to Clear the Mind 205
  B. Breathing Method to Control the Mind 206
  C. Breathing Method to Control the Body's Equilibrium 207
  D. Meditation Breathing Practice Method 207
 Chapter IX. Golden Rishi Qigong 211
  A. Golden Rishi Single-Form Qigong 215
   1. Stomach Qigong...215
   2. Lung Qigong 218
   3. Kidney and Liver Qigong 219
   4. Heart Qigong..222
  B. Golden Rishi Five Elements Qigong 225
  C. Sojucheon (小周天; The Microcosmic Orbit) 230
Part III. Qigong Practice Journals & Testimonials 243

Foreword

Sang Han, President
Golden Rishi Academy USA

In 1995, my life was a dark tunnel. The persistent pain from heart pressure and breathing problems wore me down. When I was diagnosed with a disease that Western medicine could not cure, I felt like I was on the brink of despair, at only 25 years of age. I sought every remedy, doctor, and expert within my reach, but to no avail. It was during this challenging time that Tai Chi brought light into my life, offering not just exercise but renewed hope and a path to balance.

On my first day of Tai Chi, I struggled to walk up the steps of the studio and constantly feared dying in my sleep. But I didn't give up, I kept going. In the fall of 1999, another turning point occurred in my life when a fellow Tai Chi practitioner introduced me to Grand Master Byung Joo Choi of Golden Rishi Academy in Korea. This meeting gave me the strength to dream of a new life beyond the shadow of death.

The Qigong classes at Golden Rishi Academy in Korea added a new dimension to my life, and Grand Master Byung Joo Choi sensed from our first meeting that I would become his disciple. After committing to discipleship, Master Choi invited me to climb a mountain with him. Doubts and fears overwhelmed me: *"Will I be able to make it? Will I even return alive?"*

But miraculously, as we climbed the mountain, my legs and feet became lighter. I made it safely, and the experience left an incredible impression on me. Upon descending, I immediately called my wife and exclaimed, *"I feel completely recovered; I feel so good."* She could barely understand my words as tears of joy streamed down my face. That moment with my wife was a blessed message that a new life had begun for me and for us.

Regaining my health, my family and I in 2000 immigrated to Chicago, Illinois where we began a new chapter in our lives. A sense of mission has propelled me to help others achieve health through Tai Chi and Qigong, and I eagerly wanted to share what I learned. Even though my oldest child was only six years old and my second child had just been born, I was resolute in my decision to teach Tai Chi. This choice appeared crazy to my family, and my wife who had to promptly find a job and help support our family while I pursued my vision.

During the first year, the number of students did not increase, and life became increasingly difficult. It was a true test. I began searching for an additional job. Despite setbacks, including the necessity of shutting down and later reopening the school two times during the entire process, my determination to teach Tai Chi and Qigong in the United States remained unwavering. Now after more than 20 years, with my wife's loving support, encouragement, and commitment, we have created a vibrant dojo (school) for the immersive, experiential training in Tai Chi, Qi Gong and Taekwondo.

Over time, after our moved to San Diego, the school we created has become a center for health and wellness in our community. Fueled with vision, steadfast family support, and the health principles embedded in Tai Chi and Qigong, we've established a hopeful life in this new land. People are seeking alternatives for health and peace, and we are with them. Despite the challenges of immigrant life, my passion and vision have kept my family together and has made us stronger.

In 2019, Grand Master Byung Joo Choi visited San Diego and entrusted me with the important task of translating his Golden Rishi Qigong book (published 2004) with the intention of bringing it to English-language readers. After five years of dedicated work, I take pride in presenting the completed English version of Golden Rishi Qigong. This project would not have been possible without the invaluable contributions of my students. Translating this book required a deep understanding of the history of Qigong and its connection to Daoism, Buddhism, Confucianism, and Yoga, along with a basic knowledge of Chinese medicine. This book is essential reading for beginners to advanced practitioners of Qigong, serving as a textbook to foster comprehension of the foundations, principles, history, practice methods, and essence of Qigong.

Famous Korean calligrapher, Kim Jung Hee, authored a poetic artwork titled, "Yoo Jae" (留齋) translated as 'A House of Leaving Behind'. The poetic, yet literal meaning of the work is 'leaving behind unused skills to return them to nature, abandoning rust to be reclaimed by the land, letting go of unused wealth to benefit the people, and sharing unused blessings with one's descendants.' In essence, one could say it is about sharing acquired knowledge and abundance with others. In this way, we hope to share a legacy that embodies the essence and life-changing nature that is Qigong.

This book is derived from decades of research, testing, and practice by Grand Master Byoung Joo Choi and myself. The creation and sharing of these teachings serve, in part, as an embodiment of the generosity described by the artist Kim Jung Hee. Through this, we pass down to our descendants the rich history of our Korean ancestors' wisdom of Qigong practices and training methods.

As we practice and integrate Qigong into our daily lives, we are cultivating our minds, and as we practice it becomes part of our natural daily habit. The essence of our mindset shifts to move us towards more meaningful insights into our everyday lives. This is the beginning.

Sang P. Han
January 2024

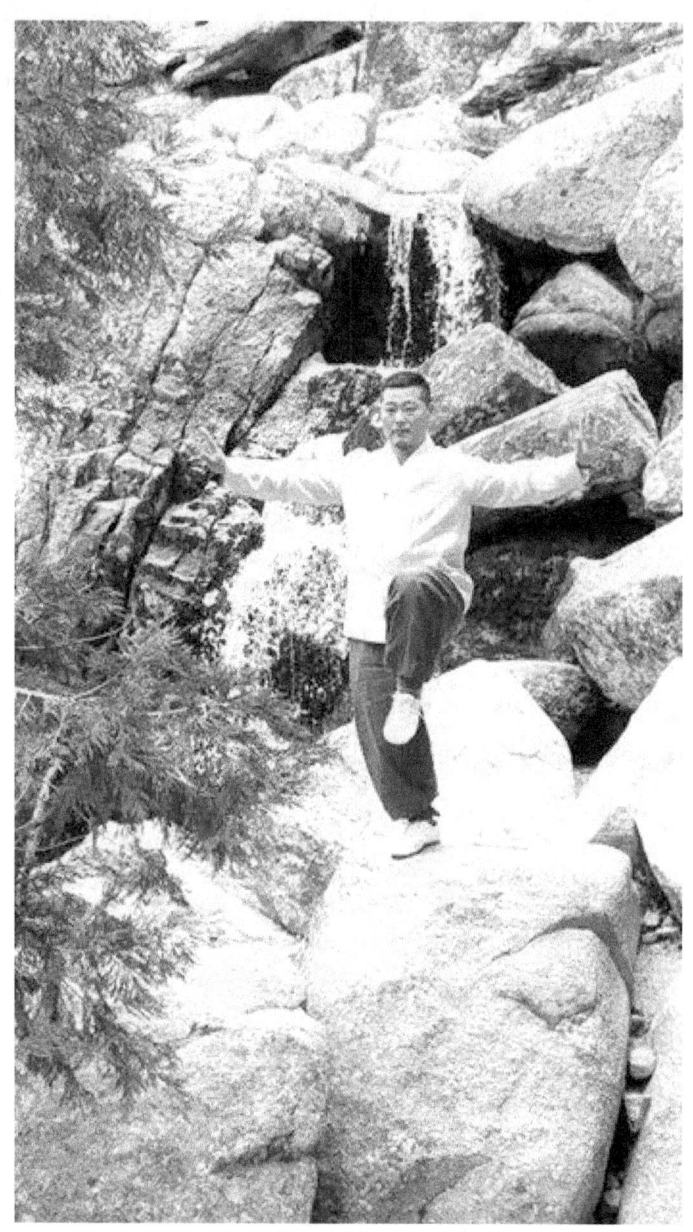

Master Sang Han demonstrating Qigong

Acknowledgements

After the initial translation, Larry Tong, Maria Tong, Youngmoon Choi, Kathy Rooney, S. Vedder, C. Barbour, Austin Gunter, Dr. Se Yong Lee and Lisa Martin came together to begin proofreading in the summer of 2023.

Special thanks to S. Vedder, C. Barbour and Lisa Martin for their hard work in further editing the book.

Further, I am eternally grateful to my wife, Heejung Han, for consistently believing in me and sharing in the purpose behind our hard work—helping others achieve ultimate health and expanding the reach of this valuable information.

Preface

Grand Master Byung Joo Choi
President, International Golden Rishi

Contemporary scholars have sought to transcend the spirit/matter dichotomy which is entrenched in modern Western civilization. The course of this quest has led them to coin the term "new science" as a means to bridge this gap and overcome this dichotomy.

In Eastern Philosophy the search to understand the mind-body connection has been evolving for millennia. Our ancestors, through the practice of Seon Do (仙道: the Immortal Way) or the through the study of the Dao, believed that mind and matter are not separate entities, but differ only in their vibrations and dimensions. They are, in fact, inseparable and interconnected at the same time.

Seon Do scholars view three dimensions in the practice of Seon Do to be the essence of life (精), Qi (氣), and spirit (神). The expression of mind manifests as matter, and the action of matter affects the mind. This understanding implies that thoughts create matter and beliefs can transform the body, paving the way for the study of Danhak (the study of the elixir field).

This perspective offers a new vision and direction among scientists, especially in the field of quantum theory. Pioneering Western theoretical physicists have been inspired by Eastern philosophies such as that found in the I Ching (周易)[1] and Seon Do (仙道). In the past 50 years, we, the Korean people, have become focused mainly on the material civilization of the West and have often overlooked the strong points of our own culture.

In May 1991, I opened Seon Do Won (仙道院) near Seolleung Station in Gangnam, South Korea, shifting from personal practice to training others. After 22 years of rigorous Seon Do practice, I have met many seekers and gained immense knowledge. My travels, both domestically and internationally, in search of excellent teachers and vibrant practice sites, have familiarized me with traditional practices worldwide. The conclusion from these travels is that all methods based on the human body are fundamentally similar.

Seon Do in particular, stood out as being systematic, with diverse practices and a long history. This distinction is its inherent qualities of the mind body connection. My encounters with Daoist (道人) and Immortals in China, often inaccessible to locals, had a profound effect

---

[1] The I Ching, an ancient Chinese divination text and philosophical work dating back over 3,000 years, utilizes 64 hexagrams representing the interplay of yin and yang to offer guidance on navigating the constant flux of the universe, often consulted for insights into personal matters and decision-making.

on me. These meetings almost seemed like destiny, leading me to wonder if my connection with Seon Do, as a 31st generation descendant of Choi Chi-Won[2], was preordained in a previous life.

With the intention of fulfilling this destiny, I vowed to restore the correct practice of Seon Do so that anyone interested could easily access it and practice it effectively. This aligns with the ancient Chinese belief in the Land of Immortals in Haedong Joseon[3], suggesting a societal transformation toward well-being. To achieve this, I began translating the most authentic and original Daoist texts into Korean, renamed Seon Do Won the Golden Rishi Academy, and opened it to a wider audience in October 1994. Despite challenges, with support and personal sacrifice, I persevered. The practice of Seon Do in South Korea, once vague and often centered around shamans, has now developed into a well-structured method. Tracing the lineage of the Dao from northeast Asia through Hwa Rang Do[4], the teachings of Kim Gagi, Jaehye Dae Sa, Choi Seung Woo, Choi Chi-Won, and continued by Kim Si-Seup and Seo Hwa-Dam, the Golden Rishi Academy proudly carries this lineage forward.

---

[2] Choi Chi-Won (born 857 AD) was a prominent Korean historical figure known for his contributions in the fields of Confucianism, martial arts, and diplomacy during the late Unified Silla period. Unified Silla, also known as Late Silla, existed from 668 CE to 935 CE, marking the unification of the Korean Peninsula under the Silla kingdom.

[3] Haedong Joseon is a term in Korean that is often used to refer to the ancient Korean state. Joseon was the last dynastic kingdom of Korea, lasting just over 500 years. It was founded by Yi Seong-gye in July 1392 and replaced by the Korean Empire in October 1897. (from Wikipedia)

[4] Hwa Rang Do means the "Way of the Flowering Knights." The Hwarang were young men or rather teenagers ranging from 13 to 16 years old who were selected from the noble families of Silla.

I still take great pride in the event that occurred in November 2000. During my exploration of the origins of Chinese Daoism in Mount Jongnam (Zhongnan), I came across a remarkable discovery. Local residents informed me about an engraved stone monument hidden within a rugged valley, nestled among sharp peaks and concealed behind a cliff in Jaogou (Ziwu Valley). We assembled a team of Chinese Daoist scholars to locate the monument, and to our surprise, the inscription turned out to be a text expounding on Kim Gagi's Dao teachings.

Upon further examination, we determined that the stone monument likely dated back to the Song Dynasty[5] and contained similar content to that found in the book "Sokseonjeon" from the Tang Dynasty. Essentially, it revealed that Kim Gagi resided in Jaogou, where he received teachings such as "Cheongwabi Mun," "Youngbopilbeop," and "Geumgoiduoak" from Daoism. He developed his own Dao teachings, disseminating them among the common people and scholars while situated on the Golden Mountain of Jaogou.

This endeavor, driven solely by the Golden Rishi Academy's commitment to contributing to national health, marks a significant step in reviving the training environment for the dual cultivation of body and mind (性命雙修) that had disappeared from this country. This is regrettably due to the neglect of physical cultivation in favor of exclusive emphasis on spiritual practice during the five hundred years of the Joseon Dynasty.

---

[5] The Song Dynasty was an imperial dynasty of China that ruled from 960 to 1279.

Finally, I deeply engrave on my heart the truths of 'Daedomusa' (the belief that one cannot attain the great path without renouncing selfish desires). I continue to meticulously refine my practice of 'Myeoljinjeong' (滅盡定: the highest state of mindfulness in meditation) and my wall-facing meditation training. When I contemplate whether my desire to produce immortals through the Golden Rishi Academy is a personal wish, I reexamine my intentions.

Byung Joo Choi, President
Pen Name: Hyunmun (Deeply Enlightened)
February 2004

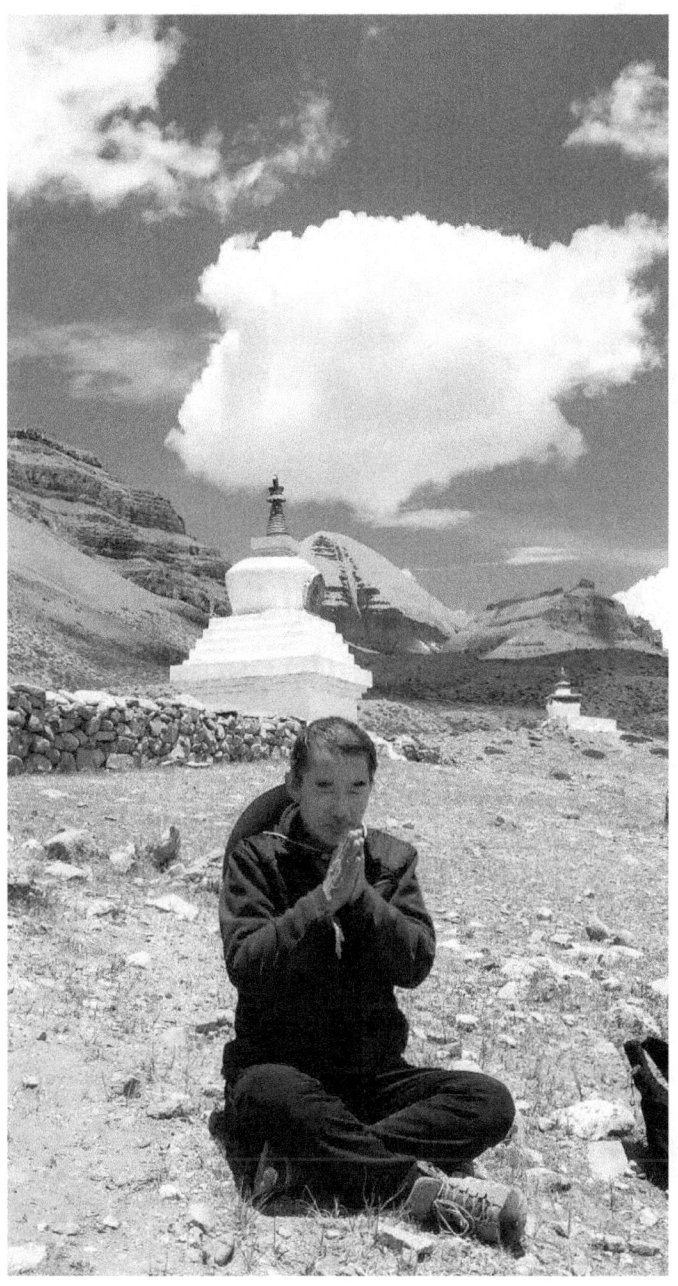

Grand Master Byung Joo Choi, Founder of Golden Rishi Academy at Mount Kailash, Tibet

Part I. Golden Rishi Qigong Principles and History

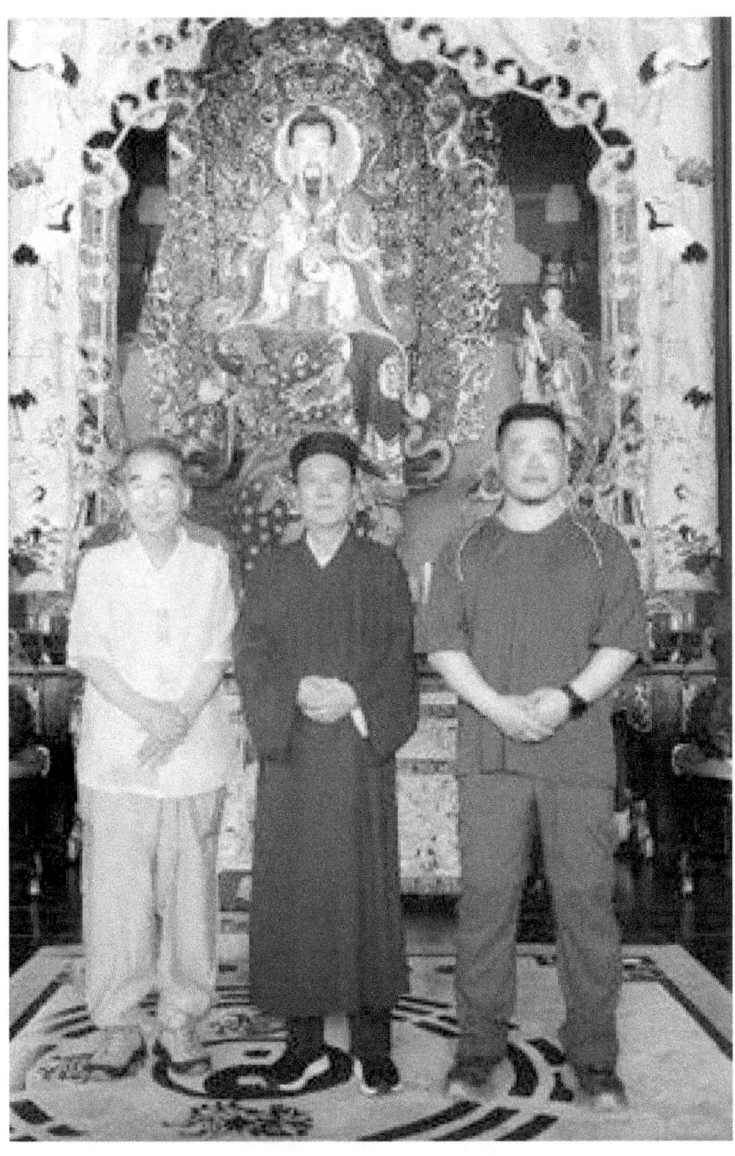

The Golden Rishi Temple located in Zhaogong,
on the eastern side of Qingliang Mountain
in Xi'an, Shanxi Province, China
Golden Rishi Founder, Grand Master Byung Joo Choi, Chen, Taoist Leader in China,
Master Sang Pok Han, President Golden Rishi USA. 2023

Chapter I. What is Qigong?

A. The Origin of Qigong

What is "Qi[6](氣)"? At its simplest, it can be thought of as energy. But it is more than just energy; it is vital life energy. Why has this concept of human vital energy gained so much attention recently? There are many factors, but it may signal a shift in humanity's focus from merely surviving to truly thriving as well as striving to reach our full potential.

During the 19th century, the issue of survival was a significant challenge for most of humanity, except for a few in the upper echelons of society. The majority of humanity's effort and time was devoted to meeting basic survival needs. In the 20th century people gradually began to experience more leisure and relief from these constant survival pressures lessened. In the 21st century, as the advancement of technologies developed worldwide, a portion of humanity now has the space in the time to seek meaningful pursuits. Many people are enjoying a healthy and enriching quality of living, believing also, that this exploration will satisfy the deep desire and quest for self-realization.

---

[6] You will find this text references two related terms, Qi and Chi. Qi refers to a general energy existing everywhere and related to the natural universe, where Chi is cultivated energy within the human occurring when practicing Qigong.

What is this inquiry regarding achieving quality of life and self-realization? It is sought internally, within the human body and mind. Thus, individuals or groups dedicated to this pursuit of understanding and refining the human body and mind began to seek out traditions that have a history in doing so. Within these traditions they discovered, by leaning on the ancients' findings, a life lineage (命脈) where the cultivation and refinement of the human body and mind are considered the highest form of a meaningful life. It is the pathway to well-being, leading directly to ultimate self-realization. It has been known through documents and records that this practice has been used since ancient times. Moreover, a vast amount of these teachings have been passed down to us in the form of scriptures (經典) known as 'Dojang' (道藏).

While many people often discuss the existence of "Shinseon" (神仙; heavenly beings), some tend to dismiss them as mere stories or myths. Undoubtedly, these beings are perceived as an ideal form of human existence, enjoying an eternal and ultimate quality of life (不老長生: meaning "undying" and "long-lived" and possessing mysterious abilities). However, the belief persists that such a life is far removed from the reality of modern people living in today's society. As a result, few consider or investigate how such beings came to be and what processes they went through to become this way. Only a few, influenced by a sense of destiny, see these stories not as mere legends, but as truths as they seek answers this world. And although these individuals have always been a minority throughout the ages, they have indeed continued this lineage (命脈). Moreover, through their indefatigable efforts, this belief has evolved into a significant cultural phenomenon. This cultural phenomenon is evident in various Qigong practices.

Many people are already familiar with these Qigong practices, and it is undeniable that all the different techniques come from a single source. This source is Seon Do (仙道), and its tradition continued in Korea, known as "Pungryudo" (風流徒: The Way of Elegance or Artistry) during the Silla Dynasty. As a result, tracing the original lineage of this Seon Do has been a quest actively pursued by all energy-cultivation organizations for decades.

There are two ways to trace this origin. One is the internal approach, where practitioners follow the teachings of historical texts and validate their own experiences through practice. The second is the external approach, involving research in both domestic and international literature as well as visiting and interacting with various Seon Do organizations in China and Korea to have in-depth discussions about each other's practice methods and principles. Through these various explorations, Seon Do practice, which is closest to tradition and most accessible to modern people, has been popularized under the name "Qigong."

What exactly is Qigong? Qigong can be defined as the refinement of the body's energy, or Chi. But how do we refine this Chi, and what are the practical benefits of refining it? We'll explore these aspects in the next section.

B. Exploring the Structure of Qigong

As Qigong was introduced in our country under various names, it began to replace traditional terms such as "the art of immortality" (神仙術), "life-nourishing techniques" (養生術), and "the art of using external forces" (借力術). Nowadays, any practice that focuses on cultivating "Qi" (氣) is generally referred to as "Qigong." This trend mirrors that of China. For example, "Golden Rishi Qigong" does not use traditional names like "Golden Rishi's Art of Immortality" (金仙神仙術) or "Golden Rishi's Art of Health Maintenance" (金仙養生術), but follows the modern language trend and is simply called "Golden Rishi Qigong" (金仙氣功). Even when broadly categorizing Qigong practices, there are two main types: the study of the Cultivation of Inner Nature/Original Nature (性功) and the study of the Cultivation of Life (命功).

Cultivation of Innate Nature (性功) typically refers to spiritual practices, such as what we commonly refer to as meditation. This includes Buddhist meditation methods such as Zen Meditation (參禪) and Vipassana[7]. In the practice of Seon Do (Way of Immortal), phases of innateness appear in processes such as Sojucheon (Microcosmic Orbit) and its extended version (Macrocosmic Orbit). Cultivation of Life (命功) focuses on the physical body, similar to hatha yoga in yoga and Kundalini practices. An example of Cultivation of Life and Innate Nature is the practice of studying one's destiny through Qigong. The

---

[7] Vipassana is a meditation technique that has its roots in ancient Indian Buddhist traditions.

reasons and justifications for this dual cultivation in yoga and Seon Do will be examined in due course, but first, let's understand what Innate Nature and Cultivation of Life is.

1. What is Innate Nature?

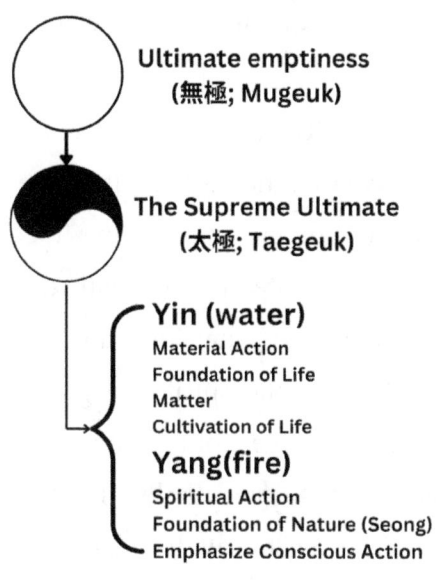

Innate nature, or Seong, (性) refers to the most intimate core of a human being. In modern times, the word Seong (性) has been misinterpreted to distinguish between males and females in reference to their reproductive function.

However, in ancient Eastern philosophy, Seong (性) means the spiritual foundation of human beings. Of course, Seong (性) is not the only thing that defines a human being, but without it, no being can have individuality. In other words, it can be seen as the fundamental force behind all cognitive activities. The state of "nothingness" or "Mugeuk" (無極; ultimate emptiness) is transformed into "Taegeuk" (太極; the supreme ultimate) then the supreme ultimate is divided into yin (陰) and yang (陽), yang represents spiritual action, the foundation of "Seong" (性; nature), and yin represents material action, the foundation of the "Myeong" (命; life).

Thus, although Nature (性) and Life (命, Myeong) can be thought of simply as spirit and matter, this distinction is too simplistic.

When you look at it more closely, it is easy to understand "Seong" (性; innate nature) if you think of it as what is commonly called "Yeong" (靈; inner spirit). Although "innate nature" and "inner spirit" are essentially the same, they are expressed differently depending on one's perspective. The term "Seong" (性; innate nature) is used from a viewpoint that emphasizes conscious action.

When we speak of "Yeong" (靈; inner spirit) we are referring to an entity that is the source of individuality. In other words, it is the foundation that allows for independent thought and action. It is separate from the whole. When this "spirit" later merges with the "soul," which takes on personal qualities, they together form a single entity known as the spirit-soul. It is only when the 'spirit' engages in life activities through the physical body that the 'soul' comes into existence. Even after the physical body ages and eventually dies, the 'spirit' does not separate from the 'soul'. The spirit provides a basis for the 'soul's' actions to continue. This is the existential foundation through which an afterlife can be experienced.

The 'soul' cannot exist without the combination of the 'mind' and the body. It is a phenomenon that occurs when the 'mind' and cerebral/brain activities interact, and it is a state that is maintained when this phenomenon continues. However, in Seon Do (仙道) the term spirit-soul is not used. The combination of "Jeong" (精; essence) and "Shin" (神; spirit or mind) in Seon Do is referenced as the beginning of individuality, called "mind and spirit" or consciousness.

This terminology continues in our language, referring to both conscious thoughts and the foundation that makes these thoughts possible. In other words, the "spirit" of the soul represents the body of consciousness, while the "soul" can be seen as the function of consciousness.

Therefore, the 'soul' is a created from the coalescence of spirit / mind activities (邪念), reflecting the birth of self-consciousness through a collection of experiences. However, the "Yeong" (靈; Inner spirit) is like the origin of the primordial beginning, where there are no such malicious thoughts; it serves as the basic foundation on which such thoughts can potentially operate. In the philosophy of yoga and Buddhism, the distinction between 'nature' and 'spirit' is even more precise.

The innate nature can be seen as the true self and is called Atman. In the pure consciousness theory of Buddhism, this is called the nine consciousnesses[8] (九識) or Tathagatagarbha (如來藏), which is another expression for Buddha-nature (佛性). In contrast, The "Yeong" (靈; Inner spirit) is not just the body that surrounds the true self; it is called Anandamaya Kosha[9]. In Theosophy, it is known as the "causal body", and in Buddhism's pure consciousness theory, it is called the eighth consciousness, Ālaya-vijñāna (阿賴耶識). From this

---

[8] Nine Consciousnesses:1. Eye, 2. Ear, 3. Nose, 4. Tongue, 5. Body, 6. Mind, 7. Manas, 8. Alaya-Vijinana, 9. Amala.
[9] Anandamaya Kosha (Bliss Sheath): The innermost sheath associated with bliss and spiritual joy.

point on, it begins to possess the characteristics of individuality and is considered to be the seed of the "Samsara[10]".

The 'soul' is also divided into two functional layers: the emotional layer and the intellectual layer. The part that plays the role of emotion is called 'Manomaya Kosha' and has been referred to as the 'astral body'. According to the pure consciousness theory in Buddhism, it can be seen as corresponding to the seventh consciousness (manas). We commonly call this the 'unconscious'. Similarly, in the Theosophical Society, this is called the 'mental body'. According to the consciousness-only theory in Buddhism, this refers directly to the sixth consciousness, which refers to our present consciousness.

Seon Do (仙道) refers to the dual cultivation of "SeongMyeongSsangSu" (性命雙修; cultivating both mind and body simultaneously) the term "Seong" (性: innate nature) encompasses everything. It collectively refers to the 6th, 7th, and 8th levels of consciousness. In other words, it includes all the activities of the 6th, 7th, and 8th consciousnesses, as well as the 9th consciousness, where there is no such activity. This comprehensive term is what's called "Seong" (性: innate nature).

---

[10] Samsara: Rebirth by Karma.

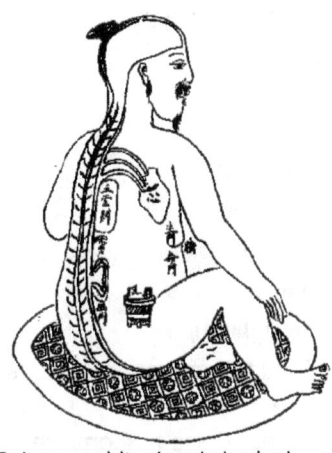

Balance spiritual and physical well-being harmoniously

SeongMyeongSsangSu
(性命雙修; cultivating both mind and body simultaneously)

Seon Do cultivation practices include silence meditation, internal alchemical meditation, rituals, martial arts, life nourishment through dietary choices, Qigong, and harmonizing with the seasons and calendar. The essence of Seon Do cultivation lies in "SeongMyeongSsangSu" (性命雙修), where spiritual nature and life fate (physical health and vitality) are cultivated in unison.

The Five Koshas in Vedantic Philosophy
Layers of Human Existence

- Annamaya Kosha (Physical Sheath): The physical body.
- Pranamaya Kosha (Vital Sheath): The sheath of vital energy
- Manomaya Kosha (Mental Sheath): The sheath of the mind
- Vijnanamaya Kosha (Intellectual Sheath): The sheath of discernment and wisdom
- Anandamaya Kosha (Bliss Sheath): The innermost sheath associated with bliss and spiritual joy

Layers of Consciousness in Buddhism: Understanding Perception and Mind in the Nine Consciousnesses

- Eye Consciousness (眼識): Perception through vison
- Ear Consciousness (耳識): Perception through hearing
- Nose Consciousness (鼻識): Perception through smell
- Tongue Consciousness (舌識): Perception through taste
- Body Consciousness (身識): Perception through touch
- Mind (or Mental) Consciousness (意識): Thought and mental process perception and awareness
- Manas (末那識): A deeper level of mental awareness responsible for self-awareness and individuality
- Alaya-vijnana (阿賴耶識): "Storage mind" or "base mind" that holds karmic imprints and serves as source of individual existence.
- Amala-consciousness (無垢識): Pure Consciousness, a state beyond the influence of defilements and karma.

Theosophical View of the Human Being: Layers of Existence from the Physical to the Causal

- Physical Body: The outermost layer, representing the tangible and visible aspect of an individual
- Etheric Body: A subtle energy body that interpenetrates the physical body, serving as a template for its growth and development
- Astral Body: A vehicle for emotions and desires, often associated with feelings, sensations, and the dream state
- Mental Body: Concerned with thoughts, intellect, and cognitive processes, facilitating reasoning and decision-making
- Causal Body: The higher aspect associated with the accumulation of spiritual experiences, wisdom, and the causal factors influencing one's existence

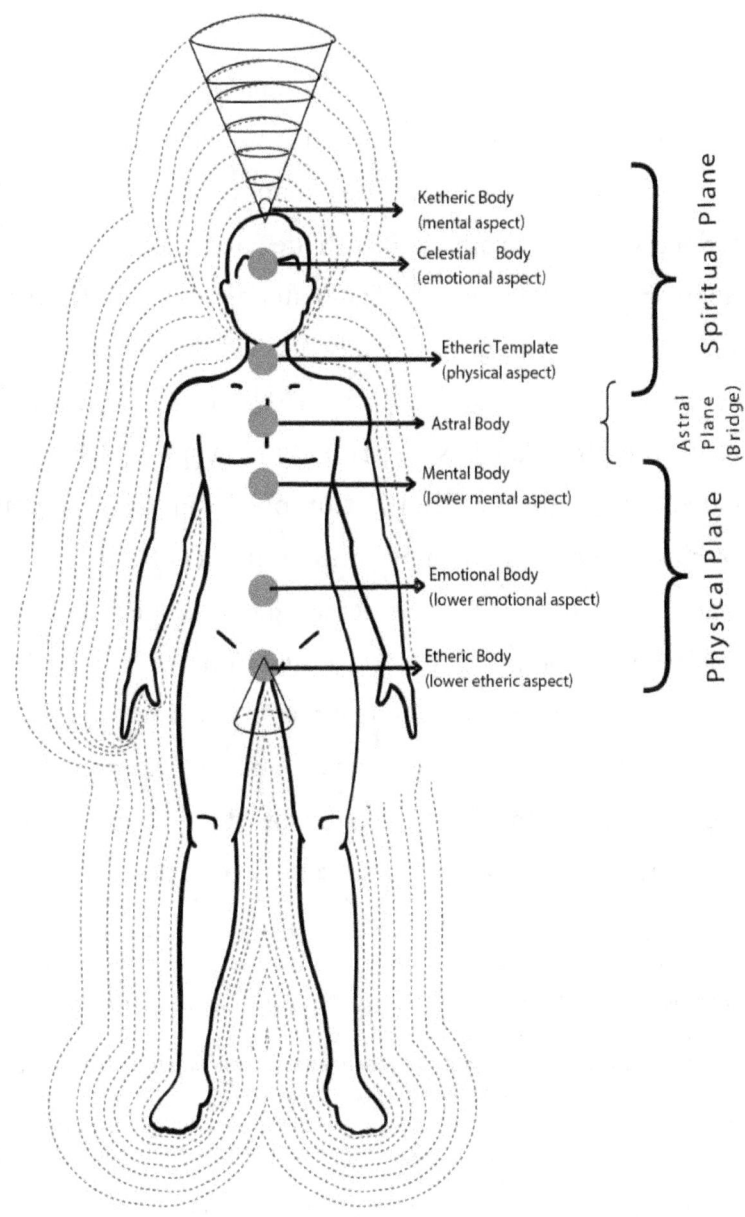

The Seven Layer Auric System

2. What is Cultivation of Life? (命)

So what is "Cultivation of Life?" In the terminology of Seon Do (仙道), it refers to a combination of essence and energy, or Qi, and the Qi refers to the living body and its life phenomena. It describes a body of material essence (精) combined with life energy, or Qi (氣). Yoga also distinguishes between the two. The material body is called Annamaya Kosha[11], while the energy or Qi body is called Pranamaya Kosha[12]. The Theosophical Society[13] referred to this Qi body (氣) as the "etheric body,[14]" often translated as "astral body[15]" in spiritualist sciences. In Seon Do (仙道), this is called the 'Corporeal Soul' (魄). Therefore, the interactive combination of a person's "Spirit" (神) and "Essence" (精) is called "HonBeak" (魂魄: ethereal and corporeal soul). When a person's physical body (肉體) is separated from his "HonBeak" (魂魄), the body ceases to function and decays. At this time, it is said that the "Ethereal Soul" (魂) ascends to heaven, and the "Corporeal Soul" (魄) disperses to the earth. Thus, the "Corporeal Soul" (魄) can be said to be closer to the physical body and can be considered a medium that

---

[11] Annamaya Kosha (Physical Sheath): The physical body, including the muscles, bones, organs, and other tangible aspects.
[12] Pranamaya Kosha (Vital Sheath): The layer associated with prana, or life force energy, governing breath, and physiological functions.
[13] Theosophical pertains to the beliefs and practices of Theosophy, an 19th-century spiritual movement synthesizing religious, philosophical, and mystical concepts to explore the nature of divinity, the cosmos, and humanity.
[14] The etheric body is an energy or life force body in esoteric traditions, believed to interpenetrate and vitalize the physical body.
[15] The astral body is a subtle, non-physical counterpart to the physical body in spiritual traditions, often associated with out-of-body experiences and inner consciousness exploration.

connects the "Hon" (魂; ethereal soul) and the body. While it is said that the soul of the deceased ascends to heaven, this can be seen as moving to another dimension. Then, it is believed that the "corporeal soul" (魄) that remains in the material dimension might retain its form for some reason and is called a ghost (幽靈). In spiritual science, the "corporeal soul" body (魄體) of the living is called an "etheric body."

Hon (魂; Ethereal Soul)	Beak (魄; Corporeal Soul)
• Often translated as the "Ethereal Soul" or "Yang Soul" • Considered the more spiritual and ethereal aspect of the soul • Associated with consciousness, spirituality, and the higher, celestial realms • It is believed to leave the body at death and ascend to higher planes.	• Often translated as the "Corporeal Soul" or "Yin Soul" • Represents the more tangible and earthly aspect of the soul • Associated with the physical body and the material world • It is believed to remain connected to the body after death and eventually undergo transformations

The corresponding physical region may also exhibit signs of weakness or discomfort as the etheric body shows signs of compromise or deterioration. For those with clairvoyant abilities, the etheric body often appears bright white with a hint of blue. While alive, its shape mirrors that of the physical body, but upon death, it loses its defined form, much like a liquid that spills and disperses when its container shatters. The subject of the etheric body is of considerable interest and research into it continues. Modern science researchers call it the "Vital Energy Body". Their findings can be summarized in the next paragraph.

The Vital Energy Body (生氣體) is composed of radiating lines of fine energy, similar to a shimmering spider web, that exist in an intermediate state between energy and matter. This web forms a distinct structure that serves as a blueprint for the physical body. According to this blueprint, nerve cells are formed, and where bundles of these nerves emerge, they correspond to the endocrine glands in the physical body that regulate bodily functions.

To maintain the body's activity, energy is constantly circulating in these fine cobweb-like lines. This occurs in short cycles ranging from three - four seconds to cycles of half an hour. Among the fine lines, those that form into thick bundles correspond to the physical Vessels, specifically the meridian channels (經脈) and collateral Vessels (絡脈). In other words, the tissues of the body are maintained in the same form because they have this life energy network. The vital energy of the body continues to function 24 hours a day, whether you are sleeping or awake. However, if there is a part of the vital energy body where the light rays (bioelectric changes) do not pass well, the physical body of that part will become weak or sick, etc.

In conclusion, the cultivation of life (命功) can be described as a practice that strengthens both the physical body and the vital energy body, and can be divided into internal training (內功) and external training (外功). Internal training refers to the training of the vital energy body, and the characteristics of these practices are that they are not fast, they are done with breathing, and they are relatively static. External training, on the other hand, is purely physical training that involves training the hands, feet, and muscles; it is dynamic compared to internal training, and its effects can be seen immediately. Most martial arts training, including aerobic and fitness training, can be considered external training.

Tai Chi can be considered more internal than external training, and here we refer to Tai Chi, which consists solely of gentle movements. Finally, internal training refers to training vital energy through breathing and body movements and increasing the energy or tension of the bioelectrical energy.

- **Shin(神, Spirit)**
- **Hon(魂, Ethereal Soul)**
- **Yeong Hon (靈魂, Spiritual Soul)**
- **Yeong (靈 , Inner Spirit)**
- **Beak (魄, Corporeal Soul)**
- **Yi(意, Intent)**
- **Zhi(智, Wisdom)**

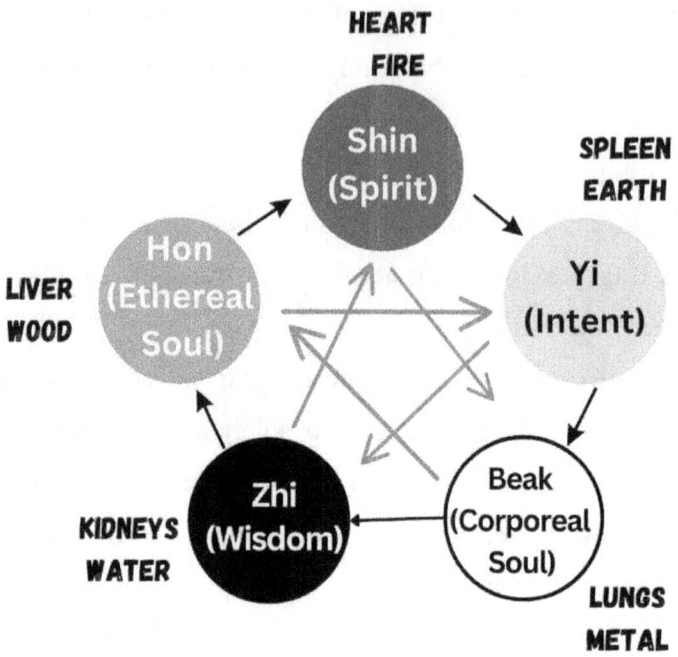

The Five Spirits of Seon Do

3. Essence, Energy, Spirit and Ethereal & Corporeal Soul

Seon Do (仙道) believes that human life phenomena consists of three main components: the essence of life (精), Qi (氣), and spirit (神). The essence of life (精) is the fundamental material of life and is the component most similar to physical matter. The essence of life is a subtle substance with a tangible quality that exists in the body and is present in everyone from birth. This innate essence of life at birth is called the "original essence" (元精). As people age, they gradually use up this original essence. As the essence of life is depleted through aging, it leads to the end of one's life, much like a battery gradually losing its charge over time. The essence of life is stored in the kidneys, and the water of the kidneys is referred to as pure essence (精水). The growth and development seen in childhood and adolescence are basically due to the activity of the essence of life.

For example, someone with a weak or insufficient 'Essence of Life' (精, Jeong) may become frail or sickly. On the other hand, if one experiences an excess of Jeong, they might exhibit a sanguine disposition. Alternatively, before reaching that state, the emotional energy associated with Jeong can undergo a complete transformation due to the effects of sex hormones, eventually being discharged from the body through the reproductive organs. Excessive mental exertion can also deplete the Jeong, leading to physical consequences such as hair loss. If one is exposed to intense stress, one may develop conditions such as alopecia as a result of the body's excessive consumption of Jeong to counteract the stress. If one's essence of life (精) is deficient, such stress can potentially lead to serious diseases such as cancer. If such a person suffers from alopecia, psychiatric treatment can often be more beneficial than dermatological treatment. In any case, all hair on the body is a byproduct of this Jeong. When the essence is deficient, the hair becomes dull and falls out. In the Theory of the Five Elements[16], Jeong corresponds to water energy.

Qi (氣) is considered a form of energy, although it lacks a physical form. It exists and has causal effects. This energy can be categorized in

---

[16] The Five Elements Theory: To grasp this concept, combine content found is the current section with Chpt 9, Section B. In this Theory, the five elements represent all things in nature (Yin and Yang principles).

three ways: energy outside the body, energy inside the body, and energy radiating from the inside to the outside of the body. External energy is often referred to as "heavenly energy" (天元之氣) or "inborn energy" (先天之氣), and it serves as the life-giving and operating force of the universe and all things in it. This is essentially a general term for all energy. When this universal energy enters our body and transforms into an internal force, it is called "inner chi" (內炁). It is expressed as "chi" (炁), distinguishing it from "Qi" (氣). This "inner chi" comes from the transformation of "essence of life" (精). Thus, a person with abundant "Jeong"(精; essence of life) naturally has abundant "inner chi." Therefore, the Jeong moves in the same direction in which the Qi flows.

"Qi" (氣) is stored in the spleen (脾臟), one of the five major organs (五腸), and in the concept of the Five Elements (五行象), it corresponds to the earth (土). The "Qi" (氣) used during the emission of internal energy is a unique form of "Qi" that contains healing power.

On the other hand, the absence of Qi emanating from a person indicates death, since a corpse has no Qi. People with an excess of Qi often have a strong sense of self and ego, which predisposes them to become overly involved in various matters. In such cases, it is advisable to channel their Qi in a way that promotes internal circulation, such as by practicing Sojucheon (Microcosmic Orbit). Alternatively, one can use their Qi in energy therapy to maintain conditions that are beneficial. Without proper guidance, intense Qi can overwhelm and fatigue many people. Although such individuals can use their abundant Qi to benefit many, such occurrences are relatively rare. This is largely due to the requirement of a very high level of consciousness in the individual.

When a person is in the womb, it is all about Qi. When a person is born it is all about "Jeong" (精; essence of life). When one practices a high level of Seon Do (仙道), human thinking activity (思考活動) decreases, and as a result one enters the state where Qi becomes the dominant element, rather than the essence of life and spirit, similar to the state of a fetus. This state is called "entering a meditative state by letting go of worldly attachments and desires" (死心入定) or "samadhi" (三昧).

Finally, "spirit" refers to the energy of mental or spiritual activity stored in the heart, and in the context of the Five Elements Theory (五行), it corresponds to fire (火). This fire, by its very nature, always rises upward. Therefore, in Seon Do (仙道), it is sometimes compared to mercury (since mercury immediately turns to vapor and rises when heated), in contrast to the water or essence (精水) of the kidneys, and is also called heart fire (心火). Within spirit, there are "original spirit" (元神) and "conscious spirit" (識神). The "original spirit" (元神) corresponds to the "original self" (眞我) and refers to the spirit (靈). On the other hand, the "conscious mind" (識神), which arises through the accumulation of information during birth and life, corresponds to the assumed self (假我) and refers to the ethereal soul (魂, Hon).

Managing this assumed self (假我) is of paramount importance in the process of spiritual cultivation (修練). One cannot directly influence this assumed self because it is the agent of all intentional actions (有爲的). It is important to cultivate without engaging in the activities of the assumed self, which is called non-intentional cultivation (無爲的). Through the light emanating from the inner spirit (靈), this non-intentional cultivation allows one to break free from the dominance of the assumed self and, in turn, gain the ability to control it.

The authentic self, or the soul that shines with its innate nature that comes from the spirit, has the power to govern the assumed self. This primal soul exists in a state of innate selflessness, beyond conscious awareness, and is aligned with a higher level of consciousness. Yet, the true brilliance of the primal state of mind is often dimmed by the metaphorical dust and grime of conscious thought processes. Through dedicated cultivation, we can purify these impurities and reveal the luminous essence of our true nature. Moreover, when a person's existence lacks this spirit, it resembles a vegetative state. To be clear, it is not the absence of the spirit; it is the inability of the spirit to dwell in the body.

So far, we have explored the Essence of Life, Qi, and Spirit. From the perspective of the Five Elements Theory, the energies associated with the wood element of the liver (木) and the metal element of the lung (金) correspond to the "Hon" (魂; ethereal soul) and the "Beak" (魄; corporeal soul), respectively. The ethereal soul is a latent spiritual feeling and an existence of material with form, but without substance. While the physical soul is an existence of material without form, but with substance. When the ethereal and physical souls unite, both form and substance are embodied. There are occasional cases where, even when the souls are separated from the physical body, they do not separate and they become a Yin spirit (陰神).

In this way, all the elements of the Five Element Theory are present in the human body. The essence-energy-spirit and the ethereal and corporeal souls correspond to water, earth, fire, wood, and metal, respectively. In this context, for ordinary people, the essence of life, (Jeong, 精) which is water, (水) becomes the center and starting point of all activities. However, for those who have deepened their practice of Qigong, especially those who are called true practitioners (眞人) in Seon Do, the Qi (氣) of the earth (土) becomes the center and starting point of all activities. If the activity of water (水) is active, positive, and impulsive, which is intentional, then the activity of earth (土) is passive and natural, and thus can be described as non-intentional (無爲, Wuwei).[17]

Non-intentional living (Wuwei) means embracing a life without a predetermined destination, understanding and trusting the flow of water, no longer swimming against the current. Allowing oneself to be malleable is about joyfully flowing wherever the current takes you.

In comparison, an intentional life (有爲的) is one in which the flow of water is unknown. Therefore, due to anxiety, one cannot just surrender to the flow. Because of this anxiety, one sets a specific goal to escape this feeling. Since there is a fixed destination, you want to reach it. However, not knowing the direction of the current, one has

---

[17] Wuwei: Non-action does not mean doing nothing or being inactive; rather, it means acting spontaneously and without effort, in accordance with the natural flow of the universe.

no choice but to swim against it with one's own strength. Swimming against it only leads to more fatigue, and as the fatigue increases, the anxiety deepens. This then strengthens one's commitment to one's goal. But the more one emphasizes the goal, the farther away it seems to be, and the farther one has to swim. It can be said that this becomes a vicious cycle. With ongoing Qigong practice, the original self instinctively recognizes the rhythms of life and harmonizes with them effortlessly. Thus, the primary goal of Qigong is not to achieve external goals but rather to discover and connect with one's true inner self. The practice of Qigong is about achieving a free-flowing life (無爲的) through intentional (有爲的) effort.

The realization of this true self unfolds naturally as intentional effort dissolves into the practice of Qigong.

The Three Treasures

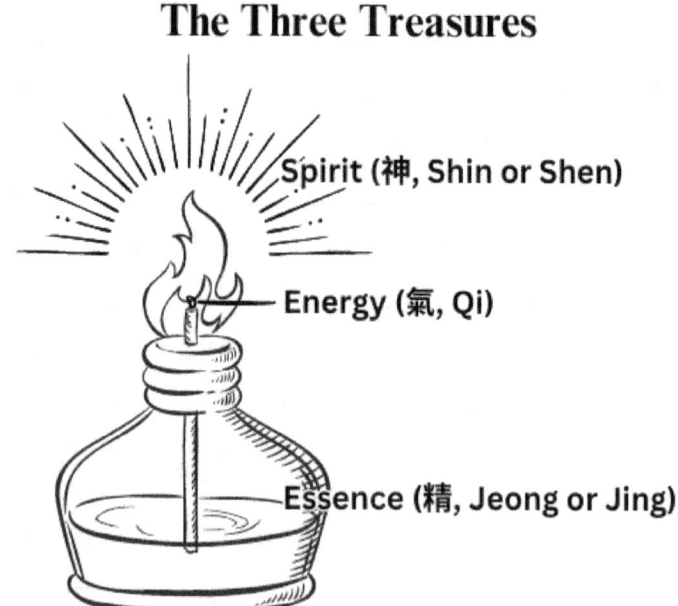

Chapter II. The History and Origin of Qigong

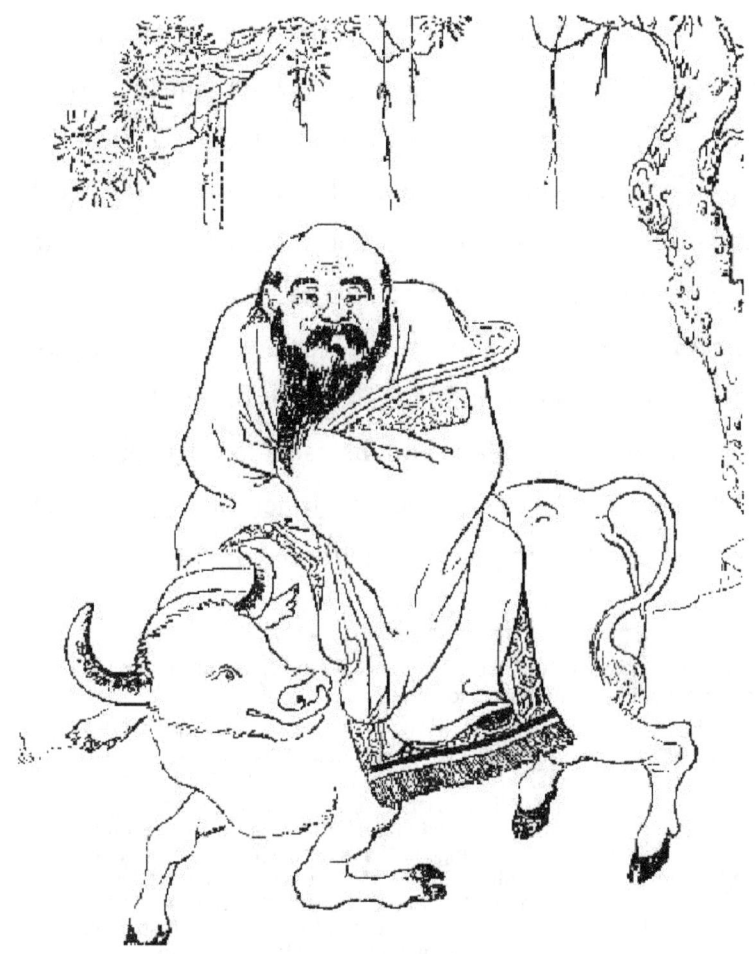

Laozi riding an ox.

A. The History of Qigong

When we talk about the history of Qigong (氣功), we can say that it is essentially the history of Seon Do (仙道; the Way of the Immortals). This is because the practice of Seon Do, also known as Hang-gong[18] (行功), is what Qigong is. By studying the history of Seon Do, we can gain insight into the history of Qigong. However, we do not need to go into every academic detail of this history. It should be enough to explore how Qigong has been passed down to us today and to understand how it has evolved into its present form.

The internal aspect of Seon Do (仙道), in terms of its specific principles (原理) and techniques (技法), is believed to originate from the ancient treatise on health and disease titled "Huangdi Neijing" (黃帝內經 aka The Yellow Emperor's Inner Canon)[19], which is also considered the starting point of traditional oriental medicine. In fact,

---

[18] Hang-gong (行功): Refers to the act of practicing or performing the skills or exercises associated with that discipline.

[19] The Yellow Emperor's Inner Canon is considered to be the most important ancient text in Chinese medicine as well as a major book of Daoist theory and lifestyle. For two millennia it has been considered as the first theoretical writings about traditional ancient Chinese medicine and Seon Do. From The Yellow Emperor's Inner Canon, we find the origins of foundations and diagnostic methods. These are integral to both Seon Do and Qigong. An important change in focus between former medical methods/teaching and the Yellow Emperor's Inner Canon (Huangdi Neijing) is the departure from the old shamanistic beliefs that disease was caused by demonic influences, and instead looking at the natural effects of diet, lifestyle, emotions, environment, and age as the reason diseases develop. According to the Neijing, the universe is composed of various forces and principles, such as yin and yang, the wuxing, and qi. These forces can be understood via rational means and man can stay in balance or return to balance and health by understanding the laws of these natural forces. Man is a microcosm that mirrors the larger macrocosm (universe). The principles of yin and yang, the five elements, the environmental factors of wind, damp, hot and cold and so on that are part of the macrocosm equally apply to the human microcosm. In fact, the theory of nurturing one's nature (Yangsheng) that laid the foundation for traditional Chinese medicine is further developed in the Dao of Immortality (Seon Do) as the practice of cultivating the spirit of immortality (Sinseon) or cultivating longevity techniques (Changsheng).

the theory of nurturing one's nature (養性理論), which is the foundation of traditional oriental medicine, transforms into the art of immortality (神仙術) or longevity techniques (長生術) in the context of Seon Do. When applied to medicine, it becomes a life-nourishing technique (養生術). Therefore, it can be said that traditional oriental medicine has the same roots as Seon Do.

Seon Do practice has been mystified religiously, while the art of nurturing life has transformed into a practical form, starting with an insight into human physiology. So, how did it split into the two concepts of Seon Do and oriental medicine? It is because of special circumstances. For example, the human body has twelve primary Vessels (正經), and it is generally believed that "Qi" flows through these Vessels. However, in special cases, there are another eight extraordinary Vessels (奇經). Normally, the flow of Qi in these extraordinary Vessels is so subtle that their existence does not stand out. However, in some cases, the behavior of these Vessels is so unique that it does not fit into a regular category and has to be studied separately. As a result, the study of these special cases progressed, and what eventually emerged is called the Art of Immortality (神仙術).

Let's first consider Seon Do(仙道) and its "Art of Immortality" (神仙術) as the original flow of Qigong (氣功), and try to trace its origins centered on literature. It is stated in Zhuang Zi[20] (莊子) as follows:

---

[20] Zhuang Zi, also known as Chuang Tzu, was a prominent figure in ancient Chinese Daoist philosophy, representing one of the key thinkers of the Daoist school. He lived approximately between 369 BCE and 286 BCE during the Warring States period in China.

"There are people who, with deep breathing techniques, exhale to expel waste, inhale fresh air, and treat these techniques as a natural part of daily existence, just as a bear climbs up a tree and a bird flies, with the only intention of pursuing longevity. These are the wise people who strive to extend their lives through the practice of the Art of Immortality (神仙術). They engage in these actions for the purpose of longevity."

It is also written in Lao Zi's (老子) "Dao De Jing" (道德經), which serves as the philosophical foundation of Daoism, "In training, one should stabilize their mind and focus their spirit. Breathing should be gentle, shallow, and long, and one should concentrate on their posture and gather their energy into their Dantian."

Meanwhile, in traditional Eastern medicine, Bian Que[21] (扁鵲), also known as the sacred healer (醫仙), talked about the method of breathing when practicing Qigong (氣功). He mentioned the so-called "Counting Breathing Method" (數息法). It is not simply breathing to get air, but a method of regulating breathing in order to enter the stage of "Deep Concentration" (入定), which is an advanced level in Qigong practice.

The documents mentioned date back to the Spring and Autumn and Warring States periods (770-403 BCE), when all Chinese philosophies were undergoing development. Therefore, it is not an exaggeration to say that the practice of Qigong started along with the intellectual enlightenment of humanity. These ancient practices of

---

[21] Bian Que (407 – 310 BC) was an ancient Chinese figure traditionally said to be the earliest known Chinese physician.

Qigong can be seen as having been fully established during the Han Dynasty (202 BCE-220 CE).

The great physician, Zhang Zhongjing (張仲景) of the Han Dynasty, is known for his detailed explanation of the use of the basic elements of acupuncture, as well as "Doein-sul" (導引術; Stretching Techniques) and "Tonak-sul" (吐納術; Breathing Techniques), which are discussed in his books Shang Han Lun (傷寒論) and Jin Kui Yao Lue (金匱要略).

Meanwhile, the famous physician Hua Tuo (華陀)[22] of the later Han Dynasty (25 BCE-220 CE) emphasized the "Nourishing Life Technique." Additionally, Wang Zhen (王眞) of the same era is said to have maintained the appearance of a 50-year-old person even at the age of 100 by practicing "fetal breathing" while lying down and breathing through the entire body by making his breathing concentrated, soft, and delicate. He also used a special "fetal breathing method" by swallowing saliva in the mouth through training.

During the Sui Dynasty (581-618 CE), Chao Yuanfang, the era's most distinguished physician, compiled all the Qigong knowledge from previous eras in his work "<u>Treatise on All Causes and Symptoms of Diseases</u>"[23] (諸病源候總). He systematically categorized these practices, making his book a comprehensive collection. So, "<u>Treatise on All Causes and Symptoms of Diseases</u>" can be considered the origin

---

[22] Hua Tuo (華陀) was an influential Chinese physician during the Eastern Han Dynasty known for pioneering surgical techniques, including early forms of anesthesia, and creating the "Five Animal Frolics" exercises for health.

[23] Zhubing Yuanhou Lun' (諸病源候總論; General Treatise on Causes and Manifestations of All Diseases)

of breathing techniques, especially within Dao-Yin techniques (導引術).

In the Tang Dynasty (618-907 CE), Sun Simiao (孫思邈), a renowned physician, wrote the extensive medical compendium "A Thousand Golden Formulas" (千金方), which consisted of 30 volumes containing detailed descriptions of Qigong (氣功) practices. At the same time, Wang Tao (王燾) wrote the respected "Outer Station Secret Essentials" (外臺秘要方), a 40-volume medical text that includes specific methods such as breathing and Qigong stretching techniques.

During the Song Dynasty (960-1279 CE), the refinement of the practice and techniques of Qigong became widespread, and it was frequently mentioned in various literary texts. A life-nourishing book of the Southern Song Period, the "Eight Section Brocade[24]" (八段錦, Pal Dan Geum), encapsulates the essence of guiding and directing Qi throughout the body using stretching techniques (導引術). It later became a precursor to the emergence of Taiji-Quan (aka Tai Chi).

On the other hand, in Korea, movements similar to the Qigong of Seon Do (仙道) can be seen in the Cheonma Chung (天馬塚) ancient tomb drawings of Gyeongju, and images of Qigong postures can be found in the ancient tombs of Goguryeo (37 BCE-705 CE). This is evidence that Qigong was widely spread in cultural areas such as China. In particular, in the Hwarangdo[25] of Silla, there is a phrase that says the

---

[24] Eight Section Brocade is a traditional Qigong exercise method that helps improve health and enhance physical fitness. There are various versions of it.

[25] The Hwarangdo were a group of elite youths trained equally in martial arts and academics. They were said to have played an instrumental role in Silla's conquest of the last of the Korean peninsula and in the establishment of the Unified Silla Dynasty (668-935 CE).

training was conducted in Myeongsan Daecheon (名山大川), a mountain stream with a good reputation and a well-known name, which can be assumed to be the training of Seon Do's Qigong.

During the Joseon Dynasty (1392-1910 CE), various medical texts describe movements and breathing exercises related to Dao-Yin techniques(導引術), which suggests that Qigong was an important part of traditional Eastern medicine.

B. The Roots of Qigong

A question is raised about whether the knowledge of Qigong is limited only to Korea and China; has it been found elsewhere? The answer to this question is 'yes.' Traces of this practice can be found in all ancient civilizations around the world. This can be seen in the term 'Kundalini' used in the broad vocabulary of India. [26] In India, 'Kundalini' refers to a high-level phenomenon of Qigong, and its origin is none other than yoga. The practice of yoga is also based on the same principles as Qigong, involving the Qigong techniques of stretching (導引術) and breathing (Tonabop 吐納法; a breathing practice that releases old energy and restores you to an energized state). The ultimate goal of yoga is a state called Kundalini, which interestingly originated from the ancient Egyptian mysticism. For example, the cobra snake depicted on the headdresses of pharaohs is essentially the same as the symbol of Kundalini awakening in Indian yoga. The lotus flower, which is still the-national flower of Egypt, symbolizes the phenomenon that arises from Kundalini awakening, where the body's energy centers awaken. It is also a symbol of an important stage in Qigong training, where a visual phenomenon appears when the Qi and blood reach a certain level. So why does the lotus flower an important symbol in China and other parts of East Asia? The reason is related to Buddhism. The founder of Buddhism, Gautama Buddha, was originally a yoga practitioner who achieved the ultimate experience of Qigong through the Kundalini process. The

---

[26] Kundalini awakening: a circumstance of the body's energy centers awakening.

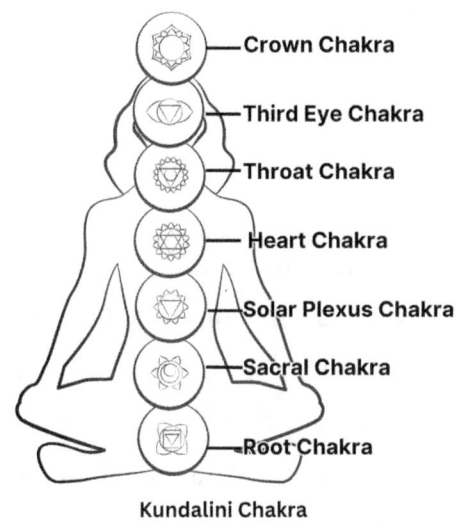
Kundalini Chakra

lotus flower was adopted as an important symbol in Buddhism and used as a didactic motif to represent how the body 'wakes up.' The fact that the lotus flower is widely known and shared throughout the East and the West may point to the widespread culture of Qigong, even in ancient times.

Let's take a closer look once again, turning to India's training methods having originated from the Rigveda Era (1500-1200 BCE). The ancient culture of Egypt once exerted a significant influence on the Hellenistic culture of Greece. All their myths and legends incorporate symbols depicting the Kundalini phenomenon, often represented by the serpent. For example, in the Book of Genesis ('Bereshis' in Judaism), a serpent is depicted holding the knowledge of good and evil, and in Greek mythology, the Caduceus, a staff with two serpents entwined around it, became a symbol of Hermes, was adopted as a symbol of the mysterious organization that Hippocrates belonged to, and was further passed down to the present day as the emblem of the American Medical Association. Interestingly, the ancient Mayan civilization of South America also featured serpents in their culture. They worshiped the snake god, Quetzalcoatl, with wings, which is essentially equivalent to the dragon in Chinese culture. In ancient civilizations around the world, pyramids and snake motifs often appear together, suggesting that they have hidden symbolic connections. It might be suggested that the pyramid symbolizes the human body, with its stone steps representing the energy rising from the spine, often depicted by dragons or snakes.

The central symbols of all these cultures, the snake and the lotus, are important marks of the process of transformation from the animal realm to the divine realm. If you go to India, you can see Indian-style statues, all of which depict a cobra snake rising behind the statue. This was their unique symbol that they were once a Buddha who became a yogi and then a Master of Yoga and achieved Kundalini awakening. Therefore, the erect cobra snake became a symbol of Indian royalty. Meanwhile, in China, the Chinese characters use the dragon as their symbol in a similar manner. Most of the columns in royal palaces are carved in the shape of dragons, which is a symbol of the dragon that flows upward along a spiral line following the spine. This represents the microcosmic orbit in Qigong. In Qigong practice, the microcosmic orbit is the most essential component, and without this process, Qigong is just a simple stretching exercise. The value of studying the history of Qigong and why it is important have already been demonstrated in the examples above. So, what exactly is Qigong, and why should it be practiced? And is practicing Qigong truly beneficial? As mentioned earlier, in a narrow sense, Qigong can be defined as the inner skill of energy cultivation used by practitioners. But does this mean that everyone must practice this inner skill of energy cultivation?

Each individual's desired outcomes and needs will be different, and there is no need to force or demand that everyone do the same thing.

Rather, we should look at what we, as modern people living in the current situation, need to do. First, we need to examine what human beings are. Using the terminology of Qigong, human beings are beings composed of inner nature (性, Seong) and cultivation of life (命; Myeong). In other words, the combination of spirit (精神) and body (肉體) creates human beings. However, the important point to note here is that human beings are not yet complete beings. The point is that the combination of the human spirit and the physical body is not in harmonious unity. Commonly said, this result is because the integration of body and mind is not achieved. Why is that? The bridge connecting the human body and mind can be identified as the brain. The brain is an analogous representation of the action of the mind. The brain can be considered a monitor of mental activities. The entity that searches for and understands that monitor is the mind. However, it is common for people to think the opposite, believing that the mind is a product of the brain monitor. It is important to clearly understand that this is not the case.

Some people commonly believe that their mental activities make up their entirety. However, if they engage in meditation practice for a certain period, they will come to realize that there is an observer who is watching all those mental activities from within. From that moment on, the meditating person will realize that the entity that they call themselves is not a mere collection of mental activities. Of course, the body itself is not the whole self either. Then what is the source from which they feel or makes them feel their existence? It is not something that can be seen anywhere in the physical world. No, the source cannot be seen even throughout the entire universe, and therefore it is something that cannot be known. Because if it were something that could be seen, it would already be an object, not a source or subject. We cannot grasp the source of 'what makes me feel?' Our cognitive structure can only grasp objects. it is like a painter who cannot draw himself while concentrating on drawing a landscape painting.

In essence, when we say, "This is the innate nature or subject of myself," it is only a metaphorical expression and cannot truly become our source or subject. That is impossible. Therefore, there is nothing more foolish than arguing about what our subject is. Therefore, let us leave the source or subject to our imagination. There have been countless expressions through the ages to refer to our source/subject, such as the idea of being limitless or boundless (無極, Mugeug), or Buddha Nature (佛性), Divinity (神聖), True Self (眞我), Existence (實存), and so on. In Qigong, it is succinctly expressed with the one Chinese character (性), meaning innate nature.[27] The Korean term is "Seong." As one's Qigong practice deepens and becomes more proficient, one can gradually learn more about this innate nature. Of course, if one discovers this nature, words cannot express it. However, one may become aware of the surroundings or periphery of it.

On the other hand, in Qigong, it is important to cultivate vital life energy (命) that corresponds to our body. Therefore, there is a subject called "Myeong-gong," or the study of life's fate. In this "Myeong-gong," there is also a practice of training to strengthen the skin, bones, and muscles, which can be commonly referred to as "Oe-gong," or external practice. In contrast, "Naegong," or internal practice, involves

---

[27] The Chinese language commonly uses multiple characters to convey a meaning.

training the "Qi" that coexists with the bones, muscles, and mind as the Qi flows through them. Of course, Qi can be seen not as something that can be trained but as something that can be converted into bioenergy within the body and well managed. This can be called "Naegong," or the internal practice of Qi energy. As a writer discovers a story for the first time, there have been practitioners of this training since ancient times who, by exhibiting abilities beyond those of ordinary people, became leaders who guided those around them. This was because they developed and used their brains to their fullest potential compared to others. As an example, the beginning of religion within a group was an idea that originated in the mind of one member of the group. Once it gained sympathy, it became a standard of social value. Consequently, society is divided into either a static society or a future-forward thinking society, depending on whether or not original thought arises within it.

Some people come up with new ideas, and some people are just followers of ideas. And in the coming times, in a future human society that includes Artificial Intelligence, who will become the leaders? The answer lies in Qigong.

C. Prospects for the Future

At the end of the 20th century, many predictions were made that caused apocalyptic beliefs to become widespread. However, from a probabilistic perspective, where probability is not only limited to Earth as the only planet where living organisms exist but also considers Earth as the average position of such a planet, humans are still too young to reach the end. In other words, humans are not yet fully mature organisms. Of course, there may be no end to evolution, but this statement refers to the current situation.

Scientists say that humans only use about 5% of their brain capacity on average, and if their average usage exceeds 10%, they are considered geniuses. If humans were to use up to 90% of their brain capacity on average, what kind of being would they become? It is not easy to imagine, but it is believed that they would become beings with psychic and supernatural abilities. The human body can be broadly divided into nerve cells and non-nerve cells. So, what do non-nerve cells do? Non-nerve cells produce the energy utilized by nerve cells. Humans consume organic matter through non-nerve cells, digest and break it down, and use respiration to produce bioelectricity. The bioelectricity generated from these non-nerve cells activates nerve cells, allowing for thinking and thus supporting life.

However, to activate all the nerve cells in the brain, 100 units of energy are required, while the amount of energy that the body typically produces is only 5 units. With these 5 units of energy, nerve cells are transmitted to the brain along the spinal cord, resulting in the brain being able to function at only 5 percent. The brain is sufficient as it is.

The problem is in the amount of energy needed that can sufficiently illuminate the dark room of the brain, which cannot be produced in the brain itself. That power source is the arms and legs; that is, non-neuronal cells must produce it. Therefore, the purpose of the Qigong exercise is to generate power by moving the arms and legs. It is not to increase the muscles in the arms and legs or to make them stronger than necessary. Of course, basic health must be maintained, but demanding more strength from the arms and legs than necessary is not required. It means that the movement of arms and legs should become a thermal power plant that converts fuel produced in the body into electricity through respiration. This is because even in the arms and legs, there are power lines called motor nerves and sensory nerves that are evenly distributed, although they are thin. The electricity travels along this power line and becomes even stronger as it reaches the spine, ultimately reaching the brain with even greater power. However, this electricity is different from regular electricity. It must be bioelectricity that is transmitted by special neurotransmitters. That is why there is no other way than food, respiration, and movement that activate the arms and legs to produce this type of electricity.

So, by using special movements, special breathing, special concentration, and even producing only twice the normal amount of power, it may be possible that one could use 10% of their brain. If more power is supplied, they could start exercising abilities that can be called supranatural because using 10% brain power is exceptional.

The society that will unfold from now on is somewhat different from the past. Due to pluralism and the expansion of individual ideological freedom, it is possible that anyone can become a leader in their collective group. Therefore, everyone must use their brain sufficiently.

In the future, many tasks performed by humans will be replaced by Artificial Intelligence. What should humans do in a world where many of the activities they used to do will be replaced? Humans will have to focus on developing their potential, which is something computers cannot do. Without developing their potential, humans will eventually be dominated by computers. Soon, not only humans but also various types of combinations of machines and humans will emerge in this world.

At that future time, humans can finally be considered to have achieved the realization of self-control. In other words, they have become a fully-fledged human that embodies their species' potential. In comparison, the current human is like a newly hatched larva just emerging from its egg. Humans will eventually need to fly into space beyond the Earth and only then become butterflies, heading toward freedom and infinite development. However, the path towards that already lies dormant in our genes. Qigong training is a method that can lead humans to their ultimate destination.

The idea that humans would easily become extinct before reaching that point seems like an invalid perspective. Of course, there is a risk that the environment could be destroyed due to the side effects of human-made civilization, but it is unlikely that humans would disappear without a fight. If that were to happen, the universe would be too inefficient. It is such an inefficient circumstance that it is unlikely to happen in a universe that can maintain its history for so long, having gone through billions of years of evolution to prepare the brain before it has the chance to demonstrate its full potential. Many scholars say the universe is moving in a more efficient direction as well, much like the law of evolution pertaining to the survival of the fittest.

So, who will be the "fit" person for survival of the fittest (適者生存) in the future world? It will not be a decadent person like the nobles of ancient Rome, but rather someone who is devoted to their development and effectively implements that development. The development of a machine-run civilization frees humans from labor, but if they spend a lot of time only indulging in leisure, they will eventually seek more stimulating fun and may end up heading toward decadence. There is much historical evidence of this. The people who have been freed from labor as a means of living, such as the nobility or royalty, have mostly lived decadent lives. If the majority of the population falls into this kind of decadence, what will happen? It will inevitably lead to the end of humanity. Therefore, to avoid the end, humans must constantly maintain a system of competition or a system that can maintain tension. As a result, for better or for worse, humans must develop their potential. So, what kind of system can be the driving force behind maintaining such tension appropriately? It will come in a form that is not an equal society, where potential gaps between classes are formed, rather than equal treatment. However, if upward mobility is propelled by personal will, achieving a free society becomes a more attainable goal.

Thus, society will transform into an environment where those who work hard to develop their potential will be rewarded. It will be a society where humans are rewarded not for the value of the tools they possess but for the intrinsic value of being human, which is their biological abilities. At that time, Qigong training will become an essential skill for humanity.

D. History of Seon Do

In general, most scholars believe that the origin of Seon Do tradition developed simultaneously among the Han Chinese and the peoples scattered throughout northeast Asia. However, northeastern Asia's literature was very limited as they were slow to adopt writing. Therefore, let us first examine the footsteps of the Han Chinese, which had abundant literature.

1. History of Seon Do in China

The practice of becoming immortal through Seon Do (仙道) was collectively known as the Way to Eternal Life and was sometimes referred to as alchemy or golden elixir (金丹道), depending on the era. While the culture of Seon Do predates that of Lao Zi, with the emergence of Daoism, Lao Zi's Dao De Jing (道德經) was adopted as a sacred text. As a result, Lao Zi came to be regarded as the founder or ancestor of Daoism.

The term used to refer to the cultivation methods aimed at becoming divine immortals and achieving eternal life was collectively called Seon Do, which was sometimes also referred to as Dan-do or Geum-dan-do (金丹道), depending on the era. Although the culture of Seon Do had already existed before Lao Zi (6th century BCE), it was with the formation of Daoism that Lao Zi's Dao De Jing was adopted as a scripture, leading him to be revered as the founder or ancestor of

Daoism and called Taesangno-gun (太上老君) in Korean. Lao Zi's family name was Li (李), and his given name was Er (耳). He was a figure from the ChunQiu Period (Spring and Autumn period, approximately 770 to 481 BCE) and was born in 571 BCE, making him older than Confucius (551 to 479 BCE). At one point, Confucius asked Lao Zi about human morality. Lao Zi spoke favorably of Confucius, stating that he was a disciple of their shared teacher. This implies that the principles of ritual and propriety (禮) have their origins in Dao. When Confucius returned to his disciples, he told them that he was overwhelmed by the commanding presence of Lao Zi, which was like that of a mighty dragon.

Lao Zi (老子) is said to have transmitted his Dao (道) to Wang Xifu (王伭甫), who was a commander in the imperial army (少陽帝君). Wang Xifu then transmitted Dao to Zhongli Quan (鍾離權), who was a commander of the emperor of the true yang (正陽帝君). Zhongli Quan transmitted Dao to Lu Dongbin (呂洞賓), who was a famous Daoist practitioner.

Lu Dongbin (呂洞賓) was also known as a Pure Yang True Person or Lu Zushi (呂祖師) in Daoism. His given name was Lu (嵒); he later became known as Dongbin (洞賓), or a Dao Immortal. He was a historical figure from the Tang Dynasty who had failed the government civil service examination multiple times. At the age of 60, Dongbin's focus shifted; he met Zhongli Quan (鍾離權) for the first time and began to learn Seon Do from him. After initially being heavily involved in Seon Do, Lu Dongbin later became a disciple of Huanglong (黃龍) in Buddhism and thus also studied Buddhist teachings, which led to him being called Lu Zushi (Teacher Lu) (呂祖師). However, Seon Do has the most anecdotes and stories about Lu Dongbin. Like Avalokitesvara in Buddhism, Lu Dongbin, as a divine immortal, was believed to transcend time and space and appear to people in times of need to save them. Ultimately, such folk beliefs can be seen as an example of the process of popularizing divine immortal beliefs in Daoism.

Lu Dongbin had two disciples. One was Wang Dewei (王德威), also known as Zhongyang (True Person 重陽眞人), and the other was Liu Chengzong (劉成宗), also known as the Haichan Emperor (海蟾帝君). Wang Dewei's lineage was called Beipai (北派), which is also known as the Quanzhen School, and his seven disciples were Ma Yu (馬鈺) from Danyang (丹陽), Tan Chuduan (譚處端), Liu Chuxuan (劉處玄) from Changsheng (長生), Qiu Chuji (邱處機) from Changchun (長春), Wang Chuyi (王處一), Hao Datong (郝大通), and Sun Bu'er (孫不二). These seven disciples are called the BeiQizhen (北七眞), or "Seven True Ones of the North."

Ma Yu, also known as Ma Danyang (馬丹陽), passed on Lu Dongbin's Dao teachings to Song Piyun (宋披雲), who passed them on to Li Taixu (李太虛), who passed them on to Zhang Ziqiong (張紫瓊), who passed them on to Zhao Yuandu (趙緣督), who then passed them on to Chen Shangyang (陳上陽). The Dragon Gate Daoism was founded by Gu Chuji (邱處機), who was famous in the Quanzhen School. Dragon Gate Daoism has been the mainstream of the Quanzhen School for over 800 years and continues to this day. Wang

Liping (王力平), born in 1949 and currently active[28] as a Daoist in China, is an 18th-generation descendant of Dragon Gate Daoism.

On the other hand, the Southern School (Nanpai, 南派) can be traced back to Liu Chengzong, who transmitted his teachings to Zhang Boduan (張伯端), who was a Ziyang Zhenren (紫陽眞人). Zhang Boduan passed on the teachings to Xuan Tai Zhenren Shi Xinglin (石杏林), who then transmitted them to Zi Xian Zhenren Xue Daoguang (薛道光), who passed them on to Ni Wan-jinren Chen Nan (陳楠), who then transmitted the teachings to Zi Qing Zhenren Bai Yuchan (白玉蟾). Finally, Bai Yuchan transmitted the teachings to He Lin Zhenren Peng Si (彭耜), who became the founder of the He Lin School (鶴林派).

In the History of Immortals, the most important figures are typically referred to as the "Five Ancestors" or "Five Patriarchs," known as the Wu Zu (五祖) in Chinese. They are, in chronological order, the Shao Yang (少陽) Patriarch, the Zheng Yang (正陽) Patriarch, the Fu You (孚佑) Patriarch, the Hai Chan (海蟾) Patriarch, and the Chong Yang (重陽) Patriarch. Their actual names are Wang Xianfu, Zhong Liquan, Lu Dongbin, Liu Chengzong, and Wang Dewei, respectively. These five individuals are considered the most symbolic and important figures in immortality practices. The scriptures that combine the teachings on immortality based on these five figures are the most commonly found texts in Daoist temples. The Fu You Patriarch refers to Lu Dongbin, who is associated with the concept of

---

[28] Currently active as of the 2024 book publishing.

true friendship. So, was there no existence of Seon Do (仙道) before Lao Zi? It cannot be said that there was absolutely none. However, it is Lao Zi who marks the precise beginning in the textual records, and prior to Lao Zi, here are some figures who existed in the realm of Sin Seon Do (神仙道; Dao of immortals) before Lao Zi.

• Chisongzi (赤松子): A divine man during the reign of Shen Nong, known as the master of controlling water (雨師), who taught Shen Nong. He is said to have practiced Seon (meditation) together with Xi Wang Mu (西王母) on Mount Kunlun (昆侖山).

• Guangchengzi (廣成子): The teacher of the emperor, who lived in the rock cave of Kongtong Mountain (崆峒山) and taught the emperor for three months. Legend says that he lived for 1,200 years in ancient times.

• Peng Zu (彭祖): It is said that he maintained the complexion of a youth even at the age of 767, and his teacher was a man from the end of the Yin Dynasty named Qingjian Shengsheng (清簡聖聖). This dates to 1600-1046 BCE.

• Huangdi Xuanyuan (黄帝轩辕): The protagonist of <u>Huangdi Neijing (黄帝内经)</u>, a book known as the foundation of traditional Chinese medicine. Huangdi was an ancient legendary figure in Chinese mythology, known as the Yellow Emperor (2697-2597 BCE).

• Dongfang Shuo (東方朔): Known for his longevity and being an expert in military affairs.

• Rongchenggong (容成公): Said to be the teacher of the self-proclaimed emperor Huangdi Xuanyuan.

- Fang Hui (方回): An immortal of the Han Dynasty era (206 BCE - 220 CE).
- Ge You (葛由): An immortal during the reign of King You of the Zhou Dynasty (1046-256 BCE).
- Wang Ziqiao (王子喬): Known as the Prince of Jin during the reign of King Yeong in the Zhou Dynasty.
- Chang Rong (昌容): Claimed to be a prince of the Yin Dynasty (1600 - 1046 BCE). It is said that his appearance remained like that of a 20-year-old for 200 years.

There were many Daoist immortal figures even after Lao Zi, but they are not considered part of the orthodox lineage of Seon Do (仙道) that originated from Lao Zi's teachings. In other words, it should be understood that Qigong (氣功) had already spread among the people throughout China since ancient times. If we list the names of the masters of Seon Do cultivation during the Tang Dynasty and the subsequent periods, we have figures such as Li Quan (李筌), Wunengzi (無能子), Tianyinzi (天隱子), Luo Yin (羅□), Tan Jiao (譚焦), Sun Simiao (孫思邈), Sima Chengzhen (司馬承禎), and Zhang Zhihe (張志和). In the later periods of the Five Dynasties (五代) and Northern Song (北宋), there were figures like Lin Lingsu (林靈□), Du Guangting (杜光庭), and Zhang Junfang (張君房). After that, there were several people, such as Chen Tuan and Zhang Sanfeng, from the Wudang Mountain sect, and the names of their schools rose and fell, but we will omit the details.

2. History of Seon Do in Korea

The beginning of the Korean Seon Do (仙道) can be traced back to Hwanin (桓因). According to the book "Cheonghakjip" (靑鶴集), written by Jo Ye-jeok (趙汝籍), a person from the time of King Myeongjong of the Joseon Dynasty, Hwanin was a senior disciple of the Dongbang Seonpa (東方 仙派). As for who Hwanin learned Seon Do from, it is mentioned in a document called "Gisusa Moonrok" (記壽四聞錄) written by Byeon Ji-su.

According to that book, Hwanin learned Seon Do from Myeong-yu. Myeong-yu is a figure who received Seon Do from the sage Gwangseongja. Therefore, Gwangseongja is considered the first person to bring Seon Do to the human world, and he passed on the Dao to Myeong-yu and Huangdi. Myeongyu transmitted the Dao to Hwanin, making him the founder of the ancient Korean Seon Do. Huangdi became the author of <u>Huangdi Neijing</u>, which can be seen as the canonical text of traditional Chinese medicine. Hwanin passed down his knowledge to his son Hwanung, and Hwanung continued to pass down the teachings of Seon Do to his descendants, including finally to King Dan-gun, who is considered to have continued the tradition. Thus, according to Samguk Yusa, even before the introduction of Buddhism and Daoism to Korea, Dao had already become the central ideology in the society of ancient Korea. According to a book called Joseon Do-gyo-sa by Lee Nung-hwa, the tradition of Seon Do (仙道) that started with Dan-gun was continued by Mun Bak, who lived on Mount Asadal. Later, Mun Bak's Seon Do was passed down to individuals such as Bo-deok, Eul-mil, Yeong-rang, An-ryu, Dan-ok, Byuk-ok, Dae-ran, So-ran, Gu-sang, Mu-gol, Muk-geo, and Jae-sa.

In Northeast Asia, Korea has long been the cradle of Seon Do. The Samguk Yusa (三國遺事) records that in the Shan Hai Jing (山海經), the ancient name of Gojoseon, Balhae, is expressed as the country of Seon-in (仙人國), and the same expression is recorded in the Yeolja (列□). In any case, the founder of Korean Seon Do is Hwanin, while the founders of Chinese Seon Do are Huangdi and Laozi.

Chinese Seon Do was also called Huang-Lao Dao (黃老敎). "It refers to a syncretic philosophical and religious tradition in ancient China that combined elements of Huangdi (the Yellow Emperor) and Laozi (the founder of Daoism), and in the early days, they pursued the goal of immortality through taking elixirs, a kind of medicinal potion, rather than cultivation techniques. In contrast, Korean Seon Do has traditionally focused solely on cultivation rather than ceremony and shamanism since its inception. In other words, it can be inferred that what Gwangseongja (廣成子) transmitted to Huangdi was medicine and ritual, while what he transmitted to Myeongyu was actual cultivation techniques. The figure of Gwangseongja can be seen as a mythical figure created by the Chinese to give legitimacy to their Seon Do leaders in later years. Some argue that there was no Seon Do philosophy in the tradition of the Han ethnic group, which is the largest ethnic group in China, and there is no mention of the Daoist in

Chinese literature or even in the Thirteen Sutras[29] (十三經) or Laozi until the Spring and Autumn Period. It was not until the time of Zhuangzi (莊子) that the idea of Seon-in (仙人), or divine beings, began to emerge, which is said to correspond to the Age of the Warring States (476 BCE - 221 BCE).

The myth of Dangun intricately intertwines with the practice of Seon Do (仙道), as vividly portrayed in the story of Ungnyeo (熊女). Engaging in a form of meditation untouched by Buddhist influence due to prevailing circumstances, Ungnyeo dedicated 100 days to meditative practices using only mugwort and garlic. This can be interpreted as an early manifestation of Seon Do. Ultimately, Ungnyeo achieved the coveted Dan (丹, or Golden Pill), thereby elevating herself to the status of a Seonnyeo (仙女, Female Sage). She acquired the ability to commune with both Seon-in (仙人, divine beings) and Cheon-in (天人, divine sage).

In a parallel vein, Dan-gun, after governing for 1048 years, ascended to divine status in Asadal. Historical records also suggest a similar transformation for King Dongmyeong of Goguryeo (37 BCE - 668 CE), who became a Cheon-seon (天仙, Heavenly Sage) after a 19-year reign. The uniqueness of the Dangun myth lies in its rarity among the creation myths of other ethnic groups, where the founding ancestor ascends to the heavens upon completing their mission.

This tradition of Seon Do (仙道), or the Way of Immortals, persisted throughout the Three Kingdoms Period. In Goguryeo, it

---

[29] The Thirteen Sutras (十三經) refers to the thirteen kinds of scriptures that are important in the Yuga (Confucianism).

gained widespread popularity under the name "Seon Doin (仙人道, Path of Sages)." Members of the ruling class with a religious inclination were often referred to as "Joi-Seonin (皁衣仙人)," contributing to the dissemination of this spiritual practice.

Legends also exist about the four "Saseonnyeo (female immortals) (四仙女)" such as the story of the two princesses of Okjeo, Danok (丹玉) and Byukok (碧玉), as well as the story of Daeran (大蘭) and So-ran (小蘭), the wives of Gija (箕子) from China, which were recorded in the Ogye-jip (梧溪集) by Yi Yi-baek (李□□) during the later Joseon Dynasty. In this regard, the Daoist religion called "Odumi" (五斗米道) also came to Goguryeo from China, but it blended well with the existing culture of Seon (仙) training without much difficulty. The fact that Daoism from China and Seon training in Korea could be well-mixed without any friction is a testament to the existence of Seon training as a tradition already in Korea. After the fall of Goguryeo, the successor state of Balhae continued the Daoist tradition of Goguryeo and widely practiced Seon Do under the name of Cheonsingyo (the Heavenly God religion). According to the Balhae Gukji (Annals of Balhae), Balhae sent a treasure chest filled with Xianshu (immortal books) to the Tang Dynasty's Emperor Wuzong, and there are also stories of a man named Zhang Jianzhang meeting a Daeryeosin (Great Female Immortal) on the main island of Balhae. In addition, Silla was also a country of Seon Do (immortal way), no less than Goguryeo. In the Samguk Sagi (Chronicles of the Three Kingdoms), there is a passage in the preface of the Nangnangbi (Nangnang Monument) written by Choi Chi-won about Hwarang-do:

"Korean culture has a sophisticated way, called Pungnyu, of teaching the Dao. The origins of this teaching are already fully documented in prehistoric records. It includes the teachings of Confucianism, Buddhism, and Daoism, which have influenced and inspired all forms of life."

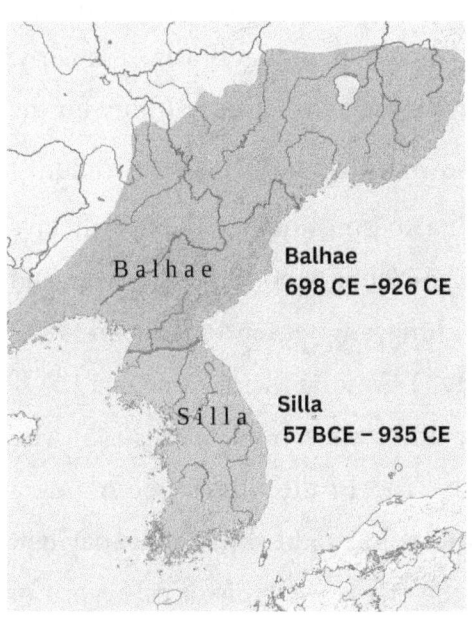

This indicates that Hwarangdo was already following the tradition of Seon Do, as it was established by the famous Shisan (Four Immortals) of Silla: Yeongnang, Sulrang, Nangnang, and Insang, whose lineage was traced back to Yeongnang, a famous divine being who practiced on Mount Geumgang. The early Hwarang organization was led by Seolwonrang, who received the highest honor as a Seon-in (immortal) from the king and his court. In addition, it is known that the famous Seon-in Mulkyeja, who was from Hwarang, taught his disciples the morning exercise method, which is a form of breathing called Dantian Hoheup (breathing). Furthermore, music figures such as Baekgyeol Seonsaeng or Ureuk were also from the Seon-ga (Seon Do Family), and the folklore of Manpasikjeok demonstrates that it was based on Seon Do tradition of music.

After the Unified Silla Period, Buddhism became very prosperous and prominent, and the tradition of Seon-ga (Seon Do Family) was absorbed into Buddhism. Some monks, as recorded in many historical books, should be understood as Seon-in (immortal persons) who practiced Seon Do rather than simply recognized as Buddhist monks. After training in the Pungryu-do of the Mulkija lineage, Wonhyo, a famous monk in Unified Silla, converted to Buddhism. Similarly, Uisang, also from the Hwarang tradition, had a strong affinity for the Way of the Immortal and was known as Jaha (慈海) in the Buddhist world. He traveled to Tang China to study under the North Five Ancestors, including Kim Gagi, Choi Seung-woo, Choi Chi-won, and the greatest teacher among them, Jungyang Jegaen Jongnijeon (鐘陵權) of the Jeonjindo School (全眞道). Among them, Kim Gagi (金可紀, ?~859) was recognized as one of the sixteen immortals (仙) who achieved the act of cultivating the Tao to the utmost, becoming a Daoist with a physical body, and ascending to the sky in broad daylight, and his story is told in Sokseonjeon (續仙傳), a historical record of Daoist immortals from the Tang Dynasty. Also, Do Seon (道詵), a monk and a master of geomancy,30 was revealed to be a practitioner of the same tradition of Daoist immortal cultivation, known in the Daoist tradition as Okryongja (玉龍子). The reason why these practitioners of the Way of the Immortal became Buddhists was due to the increasing persecution of those who came from the Hwarang class. However, the person who greatly flourished the tradition of Seon

---

[30] Geomancy: Divination from configurations seen in a handful of earth thrown on the ground, or by interpreting lines or textures on the ground.

Do (仙道) and inherited the lineage of Taese (大世) and Guryeom (仇染) from Mulkweja (物稽子) was none other than Choi Chi-won. He also translated the Cheonbu-gyeong into Chinese and transmitted it to later generations. While studying in China, he met Jong-ri-gwon and inherited the Daoist cultivation method of the Way of Immortals, combining it with our unique Korean tradition of the Way of Immortals to establish Korean Daoism and become its founder.

During the Goryeo era, the Palgwanhoe (八關會), a ceremonial event honoring the Guksun (國仙; National Immortals), was conducted. The organizers of this event were referred to as Seon Do Family (仙家). This can be seen as a legacy of the Hwarang tradition from the earlier Silla period, where similar concepts were prevalent. Additionally, with the arrival of Taoist priests dispatched from the Northern Song Dynasty, Chinese Daoism was introduced into the royal court of Goryeo. During this time, Daoist temples, known as Daoist Guans, were established within the palace complex, with Bokwon Palace (福源宮) being a notable example.

Established for the first time in the 12th year of King Yejong's reign, Bukwon Palace was responsible for managing royal events that symbolized the well-being and prosperity of the kingdom, as well as performing religious ceremonies in honor of the heavens. Afterward, the position of dosa (a teacher of Daoism) was created, and over 100,000 people were converted, with some being sent to Song China as Daoist envoys. It played a role similar to that of a national leader for all Daoist practices in the country and served as a religious foundation for the prosperity of the Goryeo royal family for over 270 years until the establishment of the Joseon Dynasty (1392–1894). Among the major figures of Goryeo (918–1392) Daoism were Kwak Ye, Lee Myeong, Choi Eondang, Han Yuhan, Han Sik, Kang Kam-chan, Myeong Beop, and Kwon Jin-in, all of whom inherited the Daoist tradition of Choi Chi-won.

During the Joseon Dynasty, following the establishment of Bokwon Palace in the 12th year of King Yejong's reign, the Shaugokseo was founded. Although the scale of the religious ceremonies had decreased by the time of the Joseon Dynasty, the Shaugokseo served as a representative religious organization to manage religious ceremonies of praying for the peace and prosperity of the royal family from a Daoist perspective and also conducted worship services for the heavens. From then on, the Shaugokseo developed into a systematized religion, playing a crucial role in the religious foundation of the flourishing of the Korean royal family for 270 years, until it was abolished during the reign of King Jeongjo. In particular, the Chojae, held at Mt. Mani (Mansan), was a national ceremony that inherited the legend of Dan-gun and expressed it religiously.

After the mid-Joseon period, when Neo-Confucianism was established as the dominant political ideology by the ruling scholar-officials, institutionalized Daoism gradually disappeared in Joseon. However, the tradition was passed down through intellectual elites who maintained an interest in it. In this period, personal meditation and individual practices of Daoism became popular, and they became integrated with folk beliefs such as feng shui and mountain spirit worship. Despite losing its institutional influence, Daoism continued to thrive in Korea in the form of a popular religious practice among the common people.

There are not many documentary records on the history of Korean Seon (仙), but there are three representative histories of Korean Daoism.

These are the Haedong-Jedo-Rok (해동제도록 or 海東傳道錄) written by Han Muoi (韓無畏; 1517-1610 CE) in the 2nd year of King Gwanghae's reign, the Haedong Ijeok (해동이적 or 海東異蹟) written by Hong Manjong (洪萬宗; 1645-1725 CE), and the Cheonghak-Jip (青鶴集) written by Jo Yeojik (趙汝籍).

The Haedong-Jedo-Rok (海東傳道錄)is the first existing record of the genealogy of Korean Seon Do. Although the book was written by Han Muoi, it was disseminated to the world by Yi Sik. The contents of the book include anecdotes about Kim Gagi, Choi Seung-Woo, and Uisang, who are Silla Dynasty scholar-philospher monks, as well as the propagation of Daoism, the path of each practice, various methods and secrets, and the lineage of the Daoist scriptures. In addition, it describes Choi Chi-won as the founder of the Eastern Seon Do. Regarding the book Haedong Ijeok (海東異蹟), written by Hong Manjong, it is a book that well illustrates the characteristics of Korean Seon Do (Daoism). Among the twenty most influential Seon Do practitioners in Korean history, the book selected nine individuals, including Kwon Jinin, Namgung Du, Kim Siseup, Hong Yuson, Nam Ju, Jung Ryeom, Jeon Uchi, and Kwon Geukjung. This book is a collection of biographies of these Seon Do practitioners, who have made a significant impact on Seon Do history, from the unique perspective of Seon Do in Joseon. In particular, it includes a collection of Seon Do cultivation scriptures (listed directly below), which is a valuable resource for Seon Do practitioners.

- Eum-Bu-Gyeong (陰符經)
- Yong-Ho-Gyeong (龍虎經)
- Cham-Dong-Gye (參同契)
- Hwang-Jeong-Gyeong (黃庭經)
- Choe-Gong-Ib-Yag-Gyeong (崔公入藥經)
- Dong-Go-Gyeong (洞古經)
- Jeong-Gwan-Gyeong (定觀經)
- Dae-Tong-Gyeong (大通經)
- Cheong-Jeong-Gyeong (淸靜經)

Finally, Jo Yeojik's <u>Cheonghakjip</u> is a collection of works by reclusive scholars who revered mechanics and folk tales, and predicted the end of the Joseon Dynasty and the transition from the Ming to the Qing Dynasty. Various inscriptions and prophetic books related to Seon Do, such as <u>Cheng's Record of Reflection</u> / 정감록 / 鄭鑑錄 and 토정비결 / 土亭秘訣 / Secrets of the Earth, were popular during this time. Novels like <u>The Tale of Hong Gildong</u> and <u>The Adventures of Jeon Woo-Chi</u> also show the popularization of Seon Do ideas among the people. On the other hand, <u>History of Korean Taoism</u> is a work by Lee Ryeong-hwa that contains all materials related to Korean Taoism and is considered an absolute contribution to the study of Korean Zen history. The original work, written in Chinese characters, was translated into Korean Hangeul (the alphabet which was created by King Sejong, the fourth king of the Joseon Dynasty c.1443). Jungeun Lee completed the translation to make it more accessible and readable to the general public. In the history of Seon Do in the Joseon Dynasty, Choi Chi-won is often referred to as the progenitor of Haedong Seon Do (Korean Daoism), while Kim Si-seup (1435–1493) can be considered a central figure in its golden age. Kim Si-seup was well-versed in Confucianism, Buddhism, and Daoism and moved freely between these philosophies. He began as a Confucian scholar, then turned to Buddhism, and in his later years became deeply immersed in Daoism. Another notable figure who moved freely between Confucianism, Buddhism, and Daoism is Hyujeong (서산대사; 西山大師), a Korean Seon (Zen) master. His disciple, Samyeongdang, also showed signs of Daoist practice, as evidenced by his activities in Japan.

In particular, Kim Si-seup left a posthumous instruction to his disciples to put his body in a jar, seal it, and open it three years later. When the disciples and monks opened the jar according to his instructions, they were surprised to find him in the same condition as when he was alive. This story is still told today, and similar stories are said to occur to Tibetan masters as well. On the other hand, in Kim Si-seup's book <u>Meuyukdang Collection</u> (梅月堂集), he explains various postures and methods for unifying the mind and body through deep breathing, as well as physical training methods. Although many struggled to understand the complicated topics written by Kim Si-seup, they were later properly understood by Jeongnyeom (pen name: Bukchang, 1506–1549 CE).

Jeongnyeom had a deep interest in the study of Seon Do, and his life was filled with miraculous events, so he was already considered a strangely unique person during his lifetime. He systematically explained and organized Kim Si-seup's Yongho Theory (Dragon and

Tiger Theory[31]) and wrote a guidebook for Seon Do practice called the Yongho Bi-gyeol (Dragon and Tiger Secret Method[32]). The methods of this practice were explained in detail and were easy to understand, making it possible for the general public to grasp and use them. After the scholar Jeongnyeom, there was a movement among intellectuals to theoretically organize the concept of "Shinseon" (divine immortality). The following individuals and their works can be listed in this movement:

• 정렴 (Jeong Ryeom:1506-1549): 용호비결(龍虎秘訣: The Secret of the Dragon and Tiger)

• 한무외 (Han Muoe: 1517-1610): 해동전도록(海東傳道錄: Record of Eastern Journey to Propagate the Teachings)

• 곽재우 (Gwak Jaewoo: 1552-1617): 양심요결(養心要訣: Essential Points for Nurturing the Mind)

• 조여적 (Jo Yeojuk: 1520-1611): 청학집(青鶴集: Collection of the Blue Crane)

• 권극중 (Gwon Geukjung: 1585-1659): 참동계증해(參同契證解: Explanation of the Certificate of the Threefold Mystery)

• 홍만종(Hong Manjong: 1645-1725): 해동이적(海東異蹟: The Miraculous in the Eastern Sea)

---

[31] The Dragon and Tiger Theory can be likened to: a pot of boiling water in the kidney/Dantien area that produces energy, the energy then spirals upward through the spinal column & spine (like a snake/dragon as mentioned earlier regarding ancient motifs), the energy then passes gently over the top of the head, then down the front of the torso with controlled intention like that of a tiger's pounce upon prey.

[32] Dragon and Tiger Secret Method: When these energies merge and circulate, one achieves a Golden Pill.

- 이규보 (Yi Gyubo: 1168-1241): 중보 해동이적(中保海東異蹟: Miraculous Happenings of Haidong Protected by the Divine)
- 이황 (Yi Hwang: 1501–1570): 도덕지귀론 (道德之歸論: Treatise on the Return to Morality)
- 이이 (Yi I: 1536–1584): 정노(訂老: Annotations on the Elder)
- 강현규 (Kang Hyeon-gyu: 1779- 1842): 참동계연설(參同契演說: Discourses on the Samadhi of Unity
- 작자미상 (Unknown author): 직지경(直指鏡: Anthology of Great Buddhist Priests' Zen Teachings), 중묘문(衆妙門: The Gateway to the Numerous Mysteries)

Meanwhile, Li Tae-gye (1501-1570), who was also known as the main disciple of Haedong (海東) and "the inheritor of the Zhouzi" (周子), published a book called Hwalimsimbang (活人心方). His book came about by studying and analyzing the book Huorinshin (活人心), a medical book of the Daoist school written by Zhu Quan (朱權) of China. In this book, various postures for Dantian breathing and detailed descriptions of exercise methods called "Doinbeop (導引法)" are included with the difficult parts marked in Hangul (Korean). Li Tae-gye, who had been exclusive to Daoism, practiced "Suryeon Dogyo (修練道教)" which Confucianism rejected. Li Tae-gye taught the method of nurturing life and recommended it to his disciples. This is a surprising event that points to how widespread the practice of Suryeon Dogyo was among intellectuals in the middle of the Joseon Dynasty.

Lee Yul-gok, who was on par with Tae-gye in scholarship, also showed interest in the Yangsaeng theory of Daoism and wrote a text called <u>Chunyeon</u> to encourage his disciples to practice Seon Do. On the other hand, Seo Hwa-dam, who advocated for the theory of Jugi, had learned Seon Do directly from Kim Si-seup and, as a result, spent his life in seclusion training to reach a high level of Seon Do practice. Although he did not leave any books on the theory of Seon Do, he left a poem about his own Seon Do practice:

"I have the medicinal properties of lead (鉛) and mercury (汞) in my body, so I regulate water (水) and fire (火) to achieve conception.

Before chaos, I met the mother of the Tao (道母) and in the midst of confusion, I obtained an infant.

The pot turns nine times, and the thirty-six heavenly realms open in order.

I am the true child (眞一子) of the Jade Mirror (玉鏡), but no one knows that this monk is Lu Dongbin."[33]

Thus, the lineage of Seon Do Daoist leaders in the Joseon Dynasty continued with Kim Si-seup at the forefront, followed by Yi Hyeson(李惠孫) and his disciple Cheonghak Sangin (青鶴上人), as well as the Seven Gates (Chilmoon). The greatest accomplishment of our people in the late Joseon era was the elevation of our national consciousness,

---

[33] Seo Hwa-dam's poem is a metaphor: I have lead, mercury, fire, and water in my body; I work on balancing these to create and then develop energy (conception of energy). Before chaos-before confusion is worked out and understood, I met the master/teacher of the Dao. In the midst of confusion, I made/achieved the Golden Pill (in a manner of fetal development). I then work to develop myself further to a higher level of the practice (true child).

which was achieved through Donghak [34] (Donghak Peasant Movement). Even Donghak was inspired by the spirit of Seon Do. However, the severe oppression of Japanese colonial rule nearly extinguished Seon Do lineage, and it was further erased by the overwhelming influence of Western culture after liberation. Nonetheless, there were still teachers who kept the lineage alive, such as Cheon-woo, Gwon Tae-hun, Mu-un, Cheong-un, Cheong-san, and others.

---

[34] The Donghak Peasant Movement was a significant social and religious movement that emerged in Korea during the late 19th century. It was led by Choe Je-u, who founded the Donghak movement. The movement later developed into a broader social and political uprising, advocating for social equality, land reform, and opposition to foreign influence.

Chapter III. Principles of Qigong

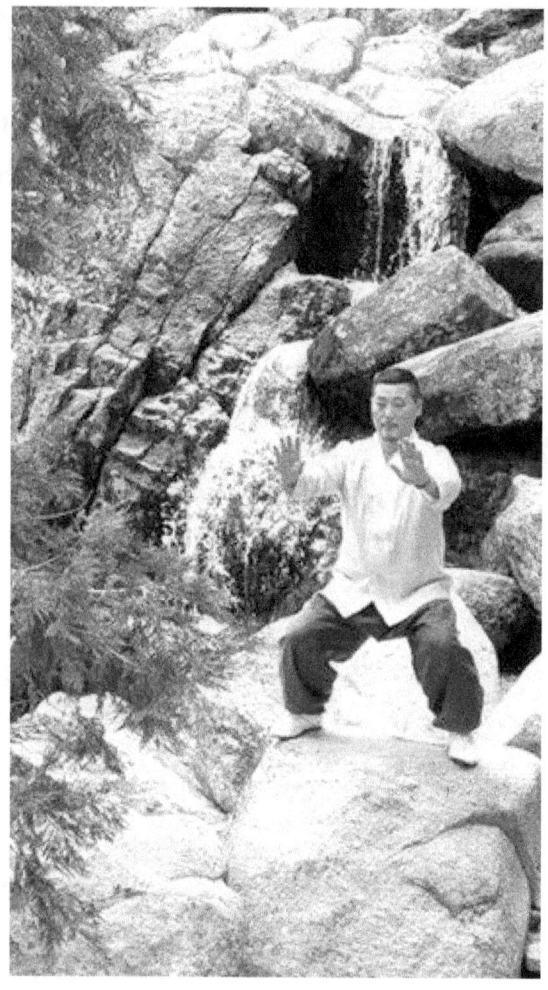

Master Sang Han performing a Qigong exercise

Before talking about the principles of Qigong, it is necessary to understand the principles and functions of energy flow in the body. Moreover, practicing Qigong without understanding the principles can be a difficult process. The practice of Qigong is more concerned with one's life than anything else, and if breathing and movements are practiced without understanding the principles and structure of the body, side effects are bound to occur. Therefore, in the past, the practice of Myeong-Gong (the study of cultivation of life) was taught only after one formally entered the teacher's school. Only under the teacher's careful supervision and protection can one safely embark on the long journey of transforming one's physical condition from impure to pure energy.

As mentioned above, Qigong comes from the traditions of Seon Do. It is important to note that Seon Do has had its share of painful experiences in the past, especially when thousands of practitioners lost their lives due to lead and mercury poisoning while experimenting with alchemical elixirs (丹藥). This history means that Seon Do has evolved through numerous trials and errors, accumulating a wealth of experience and unique lessons over a long period of time. To ignore this rich background of Seon Do and assume that merely knowing a few popular Qigong movements equates to mastering the entirety of its wisdom would be a grave mistake.

Seon Do practices describe different stages of spiritual development:

▶ Refining Essence to Transform Qi (煉精化氣) : involves purifying and refining the essence in the body and transforming it into internal energy (qi) through dedicated practice.

▶ Refining Qi to Transform the Spirit (練氣化神) : means further refining the internal energy (qi) to elevate it to the level of the mind or consciousness.

▶ Cultivating the Spirit to Returning to Emptiness (練神還虛) : means using the heightened spiritual energy to achieve a state of emptiness, detachment from worldly desires, and inner tranquility.

▶ Cultivating Emptiness and Harmonizing with the Dao (還虛合道) : refers to the process of achieving unity with the Dao (the Way) by returning to emptiness, attaining enlightenment, and integrating with the principles of the Dao.

These terms symbolize the different stages and goals of spiritual growth within Seon Do practices, emphasizing self-cultivation, spiritual refinement, and the pursuit of harmony with the Dao.

A. Refining Essence and Transforming Qi (煉精化氣)

Before delving into the principles of Qigong, let's take another look at the elements that make up the human being according to Seon Do (仙道) tradition. According to Seon Do, human beings are composed of three energy states that can transform into each other: Essence of

Life (精 Jeong), Qi (氣), Spirit (神 Shin). Just as matter is divided into solid, liquid, and gaseous states, energy is viewed as having a state that is closest to matter, which is the essence of life (精, Jeong), and a state that is closest to emptiness, which is spirit (神). The process between these two states is termed Qi (氣), often substituted with the term "energy" in general.

Even before the theory of relativity and quantum physics, Seon Do believed that matter and energy could be transformed into each other. But where does the agency that can bring about such harmony come from? The agency of such harmony is intention (意, Yi), and it is believed to come from one's innate nature (性, Seong). This innate nature is the character (性品) of the universe, and it is undifferentiated between individuals and the whole. It can be said that it corresponds to the Indian philosophy of Brahmaiva Atmanam[35], which means Brahman is the Self.

In other words, it means that Brahman, the innate nature of the entire universe, and Atman, the innate nature of an individual human being, are not two separate things. Ultimately, from the perspective of innate nature, there is no separation, discord, or individual consciousness. It is generally said that people are born with a certain amount of the essence of life (精, Jeong). The amount they are born with is called the original essence (元精), and it determines a person's lifespan.

---

[35] When the two terms are combined into the expression "Brahmaiva Atmanam," it can be translated to mean "Brahman alone is the Self" or "The ultimate reality is the true self." This phrase encapsulates the idea that the individual soul (Atman) is fundamentally identical to the supreme cosmic spirit (Brahman) in Hindu philosophy.

The original essence (精, Jeong) is a substance of nourishment, creation and birth through the transformation of the original Qi. Before a person is born, he or she is essentially a crystallized form of the original spirit energy. The original spirit gradually transforms into the original Qi, which then combines with the essence of the mother to form the body of the fetus. This is how a baby is formed and born into this world. Ultimately, the original Qi determines the quantity of the original essence.

From the time they are born, human beings consume the original essence that comes from the original spirit as they grow and develop. When they pass through adolescence and the physical body grows, this essence is only used to maintain the body.

In Seon Do (仙道), it is believed that people have difficulties maintaining this vital essence within themselves. Those who can maintain it are considered immortals or sages (仙人). All actions are driven by love or hate, joy or disgust, pleasure or anger. All actions arising from the five desires[36] and seven emotions [37] (五慾七情) are manifestations of this fundamental energy. Misusing one's essence is like shortening one's life span.

Essence of life (精 Jeong) is the base element of creation. Even those who are considered immortal or wise (神仙) cannot maintain it continuously by their nature. In Seon Do (仙道), the basic practice is to transform essence into energy (氣) and then further refine this energy into an elixir (丹藥). This process of transforming essence(煉

---

[36] 5 Desires are: Sensual, Sound, Scents, Tastes, Touch
[37] 7 Emotions are: Joy, Anger, Anxiety, Surprise, Sorrow, Fear, Thought

精) and creating elixir is considered the fundamental work of Nei Gong[38] cultivation.

When a person preserves their Jeong (精), and prevents its dissipation, they appear extremely calm and serene to the outside world. Such a person has redirected their energy inward instead of allowing it to radiate outward. This process is described in the scriptures as "turning the light around to illuminate within" (回光返照). As a result, these people may not make their presence felt strongly; they do not assert themselves conspicuously. On the other hand, those who are loud, assertive, and conspicuous are depleting their Jeong (精).

Depending on whether their essence energy is directed inward or outward, people can be categorized as either quiet or conspicuous. Ultimately, those who are more conspicuous tend to have shorter life spans (壽命) because they are constantly depleting their vital essence.

The practice of Refining the Essence and Transforming Qi, called Yeon-Jeong-Hwa-Qi (煉精化氣) in Korean, means refining the essence of life (Jeong) (精) and transforming it into Qi through alchemical processes.

So what is essence of life (精, Jeong)? It refers to the original essence we are born with, or Won Jeong (元精), as well as the digested and processed form of all the food we consume, called Gok Jeong (穀精), which provides the basic nutrients that sustain our physical body and support cell division. In any case, it takes considerable internal strength to maintain a sufficient amount of this Gok Jeong (穀精) for even a few days. This internal strength (內力 Nei Gong) is necessary

---

[38] Nei Gong: Concentration on creating the internal elixir.

to preserve Gok Jeong, which is the crystallized form of all the nutrients we consume through our diet, and which sustains our physical bodies and enables cell division.

Human beings are born with latent potential. This potential is like a blueprint of a power plant, hidden in our genes. What is this power plant? It is a mechanism designed to generate bioelectricity that could fully activate the brain. So how do we activate this power plant?

Humans are composed of two main aspects: Seong (性; innate nature) and Myeong (命; cultivation of life), which can be equated with mind and body. They refer to the method of training together with Jeong, Qi and Shin. However, this binary division may be an oversimplification that fails to capture the full picture. To bridge this gap and enhance understanding, we introduce the concept of Qi (氣; life force), which leads to a tripartite distinction: Jeong (精; essence of life), Qi (氣; energy), and Shin (神; spirit).

In the physical body, Jeong and Shin reside in different places. Jeong, the essence, is mainly located in the adrenal glands (副腎), part of the kidneys (腎臟). Meanwhile, Shin, or spirit, resides in the pineal gland, which is located in the brain.

Jeong (the essence of life) inherently has the quality of flowing down and seeking to leave the body. It is designed to give pleasure when it does. This quality is a biological instinct. Replication is the highest priority for living things. Humans, as living organisms, are naturally inclined to expel their Jeong, regardless of gender. This characteristic is sometimes metaphorically called "tiger," symbolizing its power and strength, or "lead," emphasizing its heavy and descending nature.

The term "tiger" is used as a metaphor for the tendency of the Jeong (精; essence) to always want to flow downward and out of the body, just as tigers tend to jump off high rocks. Therefore, when reading texts on Seon Do (仙道), when the terms "tiger," "lead," or "molten lead" appear, they can be understood as symbols representing the body's Jeong (精; essence) energy.

In contrast, spirit or shin (神) is often compared to a dragon (龍) or mercury (水銀). A dragon, by nature, seeks to soar into the sky, while mercury quickly turns to vapor when heated, symbolizing its tendency to soar. The energy that enables thought, essentially the electrical energy used by the brain, constantly consumes our mind through the production of distracting thoughts or worries. Therefore, the shin (mind or spirit) is depleted due to incessant preoccupation with worries and random thoughts. Furthermore, becoming ensnared in emotional attachments and perpetually draining the Jeong (essence of life) results in the typical existence of ordinary beings, marked by premature aging and illness.

Without proper practice, one cannot activate the latent nuclear power plant within oneself. In other words, one cannot awaken the sleeping serpent, or kundalini, to consciousness. So, what is to be done? There is one way, which is surprisingly simple but by no means easy. It is to make the shin (神; spirit) and the Jeong (精; essence) meet and unite so that they become intertwined. In this state, the dragon cannot soar and the tiger cannot run freely; the dragon is submerged and the tiger is crouched (臥虎藏龍), a state known as Crouching Tiger or Hidden Dragon. The meeting place of this union is the Lower Dantian, the Qi points where the secret lies. Focusing on the wrong place makes it difficult to effectively combine the essence of life (精, Jeong) and spirit (神 Shin), leading to wasted years without significant results. So where is the right place?

It is generally believed that the lower dantian is located below the navel, about three inches below the navel and one-third of the way into the body. While this is not incorrect as a location for the dantian, the term "dantian" actually refers to a "field (田)" where the "elixir (丹)" resides. In reality, the entire lower abdomen corresponds to the dantian.

In contrast, "Qi points" (氣穴) refer to a kind of "energy cavity" or "pocket" within the body, and their location varies slightly between men and women. For women, it corresponds to the location of the uterus, and for men, it corresponds to the location of the seminal vesicles. The ovaries support these areas in women, while the prostate supports them in men. This support means that they are connected to hormone-producing glands, which are closely connected to nerve cells, and thus resonate with the nerve activity of the entire body. This resonance allows for immediate feedback and harmony in response to any stimulation. Therefore, both men and women should pay attention to their lower Dantian Qi point, which is located near the perineum acupoint (會陰穴) on the meridian system.

There are various breathing methods that are effective and safe for the stage of Refining the Essence and Transforming Qi (煉精化氣).

Often, people try to get certain effects by holding their breath after inhaling. While this approach may produce immediate results, its side effects can be significant, often hindering further practice and leading to frequent complications.

These breathing methods are all intentional breathing (武息呼吸). Intentional breathing is the deliberate and conscious control of the breath. In contrast, natural breathing (文息呼吸) is when breathing is done unconsciously, without force, and left to its natural rhythm. Natural breathing is often used in deeper stages of meditation and tranquility, but there are times when intentional breathing is necessary. In the stage of Refining the Essence and Transforming Qi (煉精化氣), intentional breathing is primarily used. However, once the true seeds of the elixir have been cultivated, the focus shifts primarily to natural breathing. Intentional breathing can be used occasionally when necessary, and in the stage of transforming Qi into spirit (煉氣化神), the approach is based almost entirely on natural breathing.

The process of breathing training varies according to one's aptitude, but everyone must practice for at least one to two weeks, up to a month or two. Through this, one must fully experience the taste of each stage. This is also very helpful in guiding other people in the future because you can judge their physical condition by listening to their experiences and observing their physical condition.

In any case, as we master the various stages of breathing, we begin to regain our bodily sensations. This involves not only rediscovering various lost sensations but also gaining control over the autonomic nervous system. This process is essentially the unification of mind and body (心身合一). We cannot achieve this unification if we are deaf to the sounds our body makes. In the unification of mind and body, the mind may indeed take the lead, but how can we guide this integration if we ignore or are deaf to the body's signals?

Breathing has two main purposes. One is to create Sharira (舍利) in the dantian, which are the seeds of the elixir, also known as the true seeds of the elixir (眞種子). The key aspect here is the concentration of awareness. Consciousness is a form of spiritual energy, so it has the nature of fire, which is called divine fire (神火). When this divine fire combines with water, which is the essence (精髓) of the kidneys, it forms Sharira (舍利), which prevents the wasteful dissipation of these energies.

The second purpose of breathing is related to the awakening of the Kundalini. The awakening of the Kundalini naturally leads to the process of refining essence into Qi. There are limits to consciously striving for the process of refining essence into Qi. Although breathing can transform essence into Qi, it is not possible for someone to consciously control their breathing 24 hours a day. Therefore, if the process of refining essence into Qi can happen automatically, it will greatly speed up the progress of the practice. When Jeong (精; life essence) forms in the body, before it is consumed in any form, an automatic process takes place of refining it into Qi.

Finally, in the early stages of Seon Do cultivation, the most important principle is "Concentrating the Spirit in the Qi Cavity" (凝神入氣穴), also known as "Concentrating the Mind in the Qi cavity." This principle is essential for automatically initiating the process of Refining the Essence and Transforming Qi (煉精化氣). This stage is the first gate in Daoist practice and is the foundation for all subsequent cultivation, emphasizing the importance of establishing a solid foundation before moving forward. It is beneficial to combine this process with breathing exercises. However, it is important to understand that the concentration of the spirit in the Qi cavity takes precedence, with breathing following as a secondary practice.

When one practices breathing, a sensation appears in the perineum area. This sensation soon becomes an awareness of the lower Dantian Qi cavity, specifically the seminal vesicles in men or the uterus in women, which feels like a rubber ball or bag in the lower abdomen that expands and contracts with each breath. When the moonlight of consciousness gently illuminates this area, it is like an oyster opening its shell to the moonlight and forming a pearl. This metaphor is often used in classical texts to describe how the practice can cultivate the spiritual essence, or "sharira" (舍利), in the pouch of the lower Dantian Qi cavity.

When the Sharira (舍利), or spiritual essence, within the Qi cavity of the lower Dantian starts vibrating and tries to expand, it becomes crucial to quickly use one's consciousness to guide it into the coccygeal hiatus (窺). From there, it travels up the spine, piercing each vertebra, reaching the back of the neck, passing through the spinal cord, and finally entering the skull. This process is only possible when there has been a regular circulation of energy through the Ren and Du channels (任督脈: conception and governing vessels), known as the Sojucheon (小周天; microcosmic orbit). This orbit is a fundamental practice for cultivating internal energy and achieving a harmonious flow in the body.

The Du meridian (Governor Vessel; 督脈) usually refers to a meridian that runs just under the skin, and all of the body's Vessels run under the skin's surface. However, once a Sharira (舍利), or spiritual essence, forms, it doesn't follow the conventional path of the Ren and Du channels (任督脈: conception and governor vessel). Instead, it flows along its unique path, known as Dan Do (丹道). The process of this essence circulating through the front and back of the body along the Dan Do is called Dan Do Zhou Tian (丹道周天). The cultivation and transformation processes involved in Dan Do Zhou Tian are profound and vary greatly from person to person, making it almost impossible to describe them in detail. Dan Do Zhou Tian is not a phenomenon that happens to everyone. Attaining this state is similar to attaining a level of immortality as described in Daoist beliefs. The continuous circulation of the Ren and Du Vessels, referred to as the Sojucheon (小周天; microcosmic orbit), can result in a gradual spiritualization or Qi transformation of the body. Classical texts describe the ultimate state of this transformation as becoming a "shadowless body," linking it to an ethereal state of existence where one sustains themselves with dew and the energy of the heavens, similar to the legends of immortals (神仙) who solely subsist on these subtle energies.

It is important to note that while individuals in their 20s with abundant Jeong (essence of life) may have no problems, beginners over the age of 40 who begin practicing Ren and Du Meridian breathing techniques may experience headaches as a side effect. People commonly refer to this condition as Shang Qi Byung (上氣病) or "rising Qi disease," but it fundamentally differs from the type of headache caused by Qi rising along the Ren meridian (任脈) at the front of the body.

Most cases of Shang Qi Byung in the general population are due to Qi rising along the Ren Meridian (任脈). This is usually due to excessive holding of the breath after inhalation, which causes the Qi to reverse and rise improperly. However, headaches caused by the upward movement of Qi along the Du meridian (督脈) to the head are a result of weak Qi flow, which fails to generate a proper "condensation effect" in the head, leading to inadequate downward force for the Qi.

At such times, the Qi stays in the head, often causing headaches. Such headaches indicate that the process of refining essence and transforming Qi is actively taking place, with Jeong (精; essence) being transformed into Qi (氣; energy). These headaches can be seen as the body's way of signaling the need for new nutrition and rest due to the intense energy transformation. When experiencing these symptoms, it is wise to quickly consume protein-rich foods, pause your practice, and get plenty of rest. Once Jeong is replenished, the headache usually subsides. This process is a natural and expected part of the practice, not a side effect, so it is important to respond wisely and take care of the body's needs.

If the headache persists even after taking these measures, it may indicate that the Ren Mai (任脈; Conception Vessel) is not properly opened while the Du Mai (督脈; Governor Vessel) is activated. In such cases, it is necessary to focus on practices that open the Ren Mai. These practices involve imagining the energy gathering in the head and flowing down the front of the body, eventually settling in the Lower Dantian Qi Point (氣穴; Energy Cavity). This process can be challenging at first, but with practice, it can feel as if the Qi point becomes a vacuum, inflating and drawing in Qi. This descending flow of energy can feel like a trickling stream, or more exaggeratedly, a flowing river.

If the Ren Mai is not opened properly, there may be a sensation of liquid flowing down the face, starting from the forehead. This flow may extend down the entire face to the nape of the neck, but it may not continue and tends to dissipate. This can leave the skin of the face looking very shiny, almost as if it has been oiled.

To treat Shang Qi Byung (a condition of abnormally rising Qi disease; 上氣病), it is relatively simple: practice the four-stage breathing method while working on opening the Ren Mai (任脈; Conception Vessel) and Du Mai (督脈; Governor Vessel) channels. This method is effective in regulating the flow of energy and preventing and alleviating the symptoms of Shang Qi Byung.

As emphasized repeatedly, the key practice is to focus the spirit into the Qi cavity. Through this practice, you should be able to feel the presence of a "pouch" or cavity in your lower Dantian. it is this feeling of the "pouch" in the lower Dantian that forms the basis for various advanced techniques and further progress in your practice. Recognizing and feeling this inner "pouch" is crucial to effectively managing and directing your internal energy.

In this practice, you place your consciousness in the "pouch" in your lower Dantian. This process is similar to placing a hot stone in cold water and causing the water to boil. Similarly, when the fire of consciousness, called Li Hwa (離火), is placed in the Qi cavity of the lower Dantian, it causes the Jeong Su (精髓; essence) to "boil" or transform.

In the <u>I Ching</u> (周易; <u>Book of Changes</u>), Li Gua (離卦) symbolizes Yang, representing the fire of consciousness. The Li Gua comprises a Yin Hyo (陰爻, --) in the center, with a Yang Hyo (陽爻, —) above and below, representing water contained within fire and symbolizing consciousness. Conversely, the Kan Gua (坎卦) symbolizes Yin and has a Yang Hyo (陽爻, —) in the middle with a Yin Hyo (陰爻, --) above and below, representing fire contained in water. The Kan Gua refers to the essence produced by the energy of the kidneys, known as Jeong Su (精髓; essence), which serves as the raw material for reproduction.

The basic principle of Seon Do alchemy, Refining Essence and Transforming Qi, suggests that this essence should not be expelled but rather "boiled" and transformed into Qi. This transformation is a critical aspect of Seon Do practice, which is aimed at energy cultivation and spiritual development.

B. Refining Qi and Transforming Spirit (練氣化神)

The process of O Ryong Bong Seong (五龍奉聖; involving the guidance of five dragons directing the elixirs to the middle Dantian) refers to a stage in Seon Do alchemy in which the Dae Yak (Great Medicine or Elixir; 大藥) ascends through the body, activating the energies of the five major organs. The five organs are symbolized as five dragons of five different colors - and eventually the Elixir settles in the chest area known as the middle Dantian. This stage leads to the practice known as "Jung Seong Yang Tae" (中成養胎), which can be translated as "cultivating and nurturing the fetus to maturity."

During this stage known as O Ryong Bong Seong (五龍奉聖), after consuming the Great Elixir, the energies (Qi) are derived from the five major organs: liver, heart, lung, kidney, and stomach, and are represented by the colors: green, red, white, black, and yellow respectively. Metaphorically they manifest as five dragons. These entities figuratively facilitate the elixir's ascent through the spinal channel (丹道). The elixir reaches the middle Dantian, located in the chest.

This advanced stage of Seon Do cultivation is said to confer profound knowledge and abilities, such as foreseeing future events and understanding past events, predicting fortune and misfortune, achieving great accomplishments, or illuminating one's religious practice. This ascent signifies the unification and harmonization of the body's energies, leading to spiritual elevation and transformation.

This is also the central process in Kundalini. While Seon Do describes this state in detail, Yoga also speaks of this experience as unspeakably blissful and majestic. In its simplest terms, it is described as experiencing an overwhelming sense of bliss. And it is said to eradicate the mind of birth and death. What is believed at birth, and rooted in this world, believes in the cycle of birth and death for themselves and all sentient beings. However, such thoughts are considered to be distorted illusions.

The stage of transforming essence into Qi is a practice of transforming the Jeong Su (essence) flowing in the body into Qi. On the other hand, refining Qi into spirit is the process of transforming the Qi circulating in the body into spirit. How does Qi undergo this transformation into spirit? This stage is about cultivating the spiritual body. Cultivating the spiritual body means creating another body outside of oneself using one's spiritual energy and the consciousness of the original spirit. The ethereal soul (魂, Hon) and inner spirit (靈, Yeong) exists not in the 3-dimensional material space but in a different dimension, namely the dimension of consciousness or illusory space-time. In Buddhist terms, it can be considered a world of the color realm composed solely of light and thoughts. Traditionally, in Korean thought, this can be akin to the world beyond the Samdocheon (waters of forgetfulness), perceived after crossing the three paths of the afterlife. Of course, our physical senses, bound to our physical body, cannot detect such a space. It begins with an awareness of another world that starts with delving deeply into our inner self, beyond the veil where the five senses can no longer stimulate, essentially in the depths of the unconscious.

Since ancient times, the other world has been considered the true world, while the world in which our physical body and present consciousness reside is often considered a world of illusion or delusion. In other words, if we call the true world a "realm of illusory time and space," then the illusory world in which we currently exist can be called a "virtual time and space." Just as we refer to a computer network space as cyberspace or virtual reality, from the perspective of the soul world, our material world can be perceived as non-existent yet sensually experienced, similar to a form of virtual reality. Thus, when one contemplates and understands these two worlds simultaneously, transcendence occurs. It is at this moment that true awakening or enlightenment can be said to occur.

Therefore, if we only know one world, we are limited to seeing only one side of the coin, and we cannot grasp the whole truth. From the perspective of the other world, it is necessary to understand this world, and to do that, you have to be born into this physical world. Conversely, in this world, in order to understand the other, one must open a path to the senses of the soul, and the first step to achieve this is meditation. Meditation essentially means dimming the "Sang" (想; perception), where "Sang" refers to the consciousness created from the combination of information received through the five senses, also known as the present consciousness (六識). The essence of meditation is to dim and blur this current consciousness, thus paving the way to receive it from a different path, the soul's senses. This is what is commonly referred to as 'the inward path.' In the Daoist tradition, this concept is known as "Hwegwang Banjo" (回光返照; turning the light around to illuminate within). In other words, it means turning the light of consciousness inward, illuminating the inner self instead of projecting it outward.

Those who have completed the practice of refining the essence to transform Qi have mastered this ability of "Hwegwang Banjo"(回光返照) and have reached a certain level of attainment. They have the knowledge and ability to create a body in the dimension that corresponds to this state. This process involves refining a person's Jeong (精; essence) into Qi (氣; energy) and then using this Qi to enter the world of ultimate peace, nurturing and growing the soul body in that realm. Cultivating this soul body, which is essentially spirit, is the essence of refining Qi to transform into spirit. This practice involves the transformation of three energy elements—Jeong (essence of life), Qi (energy), and Shin (spirit)—to create a new form of spiritual energy.

In contrast to the more physical body work done earlier, one's imagination heavily influences this stage of the practice. When one connects to one's own imagination space, or, in other words, contacts the sensory pathways of the soul and enters that space, one's unconscious imagination unfolds with a realism that can surpass actual reality. This space is a spiritual dimension. However, it is important to note that the initial stage of this spiritual dimension still overlaps with the physical world.

Various beings inhabit this intermediate state of existence between death and rebirth in another world. One must be careful not to get trapped in this spirit world, which can become a demonic realm (魔境). Once a demonic realm captures someone, it dominates their thought processes. This causes significant changes and effects in daily life, making normal life difficult after awakening. This is similar to the typical symptoms of schizophrenia, where the distinction between illusion and reality becomes blurred. Venturing into the inner realms without having purified one's desires, fears, and various emotions can be undesirable and lead to problematic results. To illustrate how things can get distorted, it is like a person who needs to cross from one side of the street to the other but becomes so engrossed in the fascinating and amusing sights within an underground passageway that one forgets the original purpose for descending into the tunnel. As a result, one may begin to believe that the underground world is the real one, not realizing that the beings one encounters there are either products of the imagination or manifestations of fears. One may begin to view these entities as objectively real beings, worthy of faith and belief. It is a concern that immersing oneself solely in one's prejudices and dogmas can lead others astray, possibly to extremism. This happens when we live in a narrow world and believe only in our own convictions.

When discussing Qigong, it may seem that meditation is overemphasized, but in reality, Qigong and meditation are like two sides of the same coin; neither can exist without the other. While many people think that practicing meditation means there's no need for Qigong, the truth is that the mind cannot exist without the body, and vice versa. Although there's a lot of emphasis on the state of "Mushim" (no mind), this refers to a specific moment or dimension and is a unique experience. Therefore, a more realistic expression would be 'Hansim' (idle mind) rather than 'Mushim'.

Hansim (閑心) refers to a state of mind that is free from the complications of desire and constant pursuit, leading to a simpler way of life. In such a lifestyle, one can feel the harmony and balance between one's body and the natural energy around them. This awareness and awakening to such sensations are essentially what Qigong is about. It is a life of understanding and experiencing through the body.

Most modern people understand life with their heads, especially if one does not live in the countryside. Urban life is primarily about receiving and processing everything with the head, which becomes the mainstay of existence. Only on special vacations in nature do we find the leisure to feel something with our bodies, but such opportunities are not easy to obtain. Qigong, on the other hand, is about awakening the body's senses and knowing nature and the environment through the body. The medium of this knowledge is Qi. In a world made of Qi, knowing Qi means deeper understanding of everything. Just like connecting to cyberspace, connecting to Qi allows one to understand the world of Qi.

The "Qi" energy world exists as information before it is translated through the five senses. When this energy world is received as information by our brain, we translate it into sound or form and accept it. We understand the physical world through the five senses. Interpreting the energy world is not an easy task. However, through a long period of training in Qi energy, a practitioner can create one's own path that can also be helpful to others.

The stage of "Yeon-Gi-Hwa-Shin" (鍊氣化神), which is the Refining Qi and Transforming Spirit, is a high level of Qi energy practice. From the perspective of Seon Do, the Dae Dan (大丹; Great Elixir) placed in the heart serves as the material for the construction of the spiritual body (養神, Yang Shin). At this stage, the original soul (元神, Won Shin) becomes the spirit soul of the spiritual body. In other words, the body is essentially active energy, while the spirit soul is related to the functions of consciousness. The emergence of a spirit soul in the spiritual body signifies the development of a center of consciousness in the heart.

People who do not practice spiritual disciplines usually have their consciousness confined to their minds. However, when you practice Yang Shin (spiritual body) cultivation, a new center of consciousness can develop in your heart. This center of consciousness in the heart transcends space and time and grants what is known as "clairvoyance." Clairvoyance is not a spatial concept. It implies illusionary space and extrasensory perception that is not necessarily discerned through the human senses. Every person's spiritual body (靈體) and soul body (魂體) inherently possess such ability. The problem is that the apparatus of our current consciousness (六識) is so strong that it doesn't recognize anything else, and that hinders further development.

Regardless, the key aspect in this stage, namely the Yangtai (養胎) cultivation process, is to immerse oneself in deep meditation (大定). In this state, the Qi ascending through the governor vessel turns into Jade Elixir[39](玉液) in the center of the head. Because of the profound depth of meditation, this Jade Elixir is further transformed into an even higher-quality Golden Elixir (金液). This Golden Elixir becomes the energy that nourishes the Spiritual Body (養神). The naturally occurring ascent through the governor vessel and descent through the conception vessel means that there's no need to consciously control one's breathing. In fact, from this stage on, all the exercises involve natural breathing. One should completely forget about breathing and focus only on the bright Great Elixir (大丹) in the heart.

This refers to a state in which external objects are forgotten, the senses are dormant, and only consciousness remains awake. In Buddhism, this state is called "fully awake yet fully tranquil" (醒醒寂

---

[39] Jade Elixir is a mystical substance in Taoist alchemy symbolizing immortality and spiritual refinement. It represents the essence of life and the cultivation of vital energy through practices like meditation and breathing exercises

寂). This is the ideal state of meditation, which exists at the boundary between waking and sleeping. It is at this boundary that transcendence occurs. It is not a matter of choosing one side or the other, but of observing both simultaneously from the boundary line. It is in this observation that a new, profound understanding unfolds.

In this state, the mind no longer succumbs to worldly desires, allowing for the union of shin (神; spirit) and Qi (氣; energy). This union can be described as the fusion of innate nature (性) and life purpose (命). As a result of this fusion, the Qi of the five major organs are revitalized, rejuvenating the body and nourishing the immortal body (聖胎). At this stage, one feels like being in a state of chaos, where the new Qi is being reborn. From this point on, the five energies of green, red, black, white, and yellow emerge from the liver, heart, kidney, lungs, and spleen, respectively, and ascend to the crown of the head. In Seon Do, this phenomenon is specifically referred to as "the cultivation of the energy of the five major organs up to the crown of the head," known as "O Gi Cho Won (五氣朝元)," which differs from "Oh Ryong Bong Seong (五龍奉聖)" – involving the guidance of five dragons directing the elixirs to the middle Dantian. "O Gi Cho Won (五氣朝元) emphasized the harmonization and elevation of the five organ energies. Aligning them with the Dao, while "Oh Ryong Bong Seong (五龍奉聖)" focuses on the symbolic journey of the elixir guided by five dragons, representing the ascent of refined energies to a specific spiritual center.

During this process, the Essence of Life (Jeong, 精), Energy (Qi, 氣), and Spirit (Shin, 神) in the body are further refined into the forms of the Lead Flower (鉛花), Silver Flower (銀花), and Gold Flower (金花) flowing along the governor vessel. This state is called Samhwa Chujeong (三花聚頂), which means the "convergence of the three flowers at the crown of the head." In Samhwa Chujeong, the colors of each flower change according to the depth of an individual's spiritual cultivation. Initially, they show the acquired Qi colors of red, blue, and black, which gradually transform into the pure and unadulterated innate Qi colors of red golden light (赤金光), white golden light (白金光), and purple golden light (紫金光).

As this phenomenon continues, the body begins to undergo a fundamental change in its constitution. During this process, the accumulated impurities from food begin to be expelled from the body, a state that can be extremely unpleasant to endure. However, one must not be alarmed and must continue to meditate deeply. At some point, altars of Lotus Flowers will appear in the upper, middle, and lower Dantian, and you may see an image of a child sitting cross-legged on these altars. This illusion arises from the formation of the Qi framework of the elixir (丹) and should not interrupt one's mind or concentration.

During the silver and gold waves, an illusion may appear of a red snake traveling through the body and entering the spine through the coccygeal gate. This snake then ascends the spine and enters the head. This phenomenon symbolizes the innate Qi (先天氣) transforming into the original essence to nourish the elixir in the body. A similar process is often described in Kundalini practices. When the snake appears red, it represents the acquired essence of Qi. When it glows with the light of red gold, it indicates the transformation of innate Qi into its original essence.

While the acquired essence derived from the grain essence (穀精) is an energy produced within the body, the innate Qi is a purer and more refined energy that is drawn from the outside through breathing. This original essence, regardless of its quantity, does not arouse sensual desires, unlike the acquired essence, which, when abundant, can stimulate hormones and arouse desires. In the early stages of Seon Do cultivation, especially in the phase of refining the essence into energy, this acquired essence must be transformed through breathing exercises. However, in the later stage of "refining energy into spirit," this form of essence no longer arises.

Even without practicing Byeok Gok (辟穀; grain fasting) or following a strict diet, the body and mind reach a state of purity and simplicity where the cloudy essence (濁精) is no longer produced and the Essence of Life (精) is instantly and automatically transformed into energy. When the body stops producing grain essence, the sensitivity of perception and consciousness becomes extremely heightened, making it difficult for such individuals to live among ordinary people in a polluted world. They are often forced to retreat to a quiet, rural environment.

To cultivate the spiritual embryo (養胎), the innate Qi is not only transformed into the original essence but also spiritual fire (神火), which is visualized as the sun. This process, similar to the image of the red snake, roams throughout the body, piercing the Vessels and channels of the Qi points and appearing like countless flaming arrows. If one remains detached and simply observes, a spectacle of light emanating from every pore of the body will unfold. When one's practice reaches this level, the conscious spirit, once the ego, loses its former tendencies and transforms into a protective spirit (護法神) that actively assists the cultivation process. This is where the subtle workings of "unconscious help" come into play.

As the Dan (丹; elixir) located in the chest matures, the power of the mind becomes so strong that it can quickly cause changes in the body. In other words, a sense of control over the autonomic nervous system develops. For example, if one wants to generate heat in the body, the heat of the Dantian will quickly rise and envelop the body in a fiery glow. In such cases, it is imperative to immediately visualize the black turtle, a symbol of Water Energy. Delaying this visualization risks burning the Dan (丹, elixir). When the black turtle is visualized, it emits an icy coldness that cools the intense heat.

During the stage of refining the essence into Qi, the body develops a cooling and heating system far more powerful than the Ida and Pingala pathways in traditional yogic systems although this is essentially an upgraded version of Ida and Pingala. Meanwhile, various delusive demons often appear in dreams or illusions. At such times, one should not allow one's mind to be disturbed; instead, these demons can be completely incinerated with fire. This fire rises from one's Dantian along the Renmai (Conception Vessel) and exits through the mouth, and it is important to note that one's Dantian is connected to the sun outside the body. If a practitioner dreams or sees visions of a fire breaking out in his house or a flood occurring, this indicates an imbalance between heat and cold internally, with one element overpowering the other. Instead of causing emotional turmoil, one can either observe the Black Turtle of the moon or contemplate the White Turtle of the Sun to regulate the body's temperature. Severe mental disturbances can lead to a miscarriage of the spiritual process. Miscarriage here means failing to cultivate the "Yangshin" (養神; spiritual body), which may lead to the formation of a "Yinshin" (陰神; shadow spirit) instead. There's a saying that if you give birth to a "Yinshin" (陰神; shadow spirit), you won't be able to become a heavenly immortal (天仙) after you die, but instead you'll become a "Guiseon" (鬼仙; ghostly immortal). Although being a Guiseon[40] is very different from the state of ordinary beings, it is not the same as reaching the heights of heavenly immortality.

The practice at this stage involves not only the cultivation of the Dan (丹; Elixir) or "YangTai" (養胎; nurturing the fetus), but also, crucially, the release of the Dan outside the body. An essential part of this process is opening the crown gate (百會), also known as opening the heavenly gate (開天門). Opening the crown gate (百會, Baeghoe) is like melting iron with fire; it involves using the inner and outer fires of the body. It is important not to be frightened by the feeling of the skull cracking or the intense burning pain that can accompany the opening of this gate. In fact, the more intense the pain, the faster the process tends to be. Some people, often because they let it happen without doing anything, experience a delay in the opening of the crown gate (百會). For such individuals, it may be helpful to visualize piercing their skull with an oxyacetylene welding torch. Once the

---

[40] Guiseon (鬼仙): the lowest rank among the Five Immortals, and its appearance is uncertain, so it cannot be named in either the underworld or the divine world. While ordinary people experience reincarnation after death, a Guiseon cannot.

crown gate is open, the "Yangshin" (養神; spiritual body) can be released, marking the beginning of the next stage of the practice.

C. Cultivating the Spirit and Returning to Emptiness (練神還虛)

The concept of transforming Shin (神, spirit) into emptiness refers to transcending the limitations of the spiritual body beyond the dimensions of physical space. It involves a practice in which space becomes Yangshin (spiritual body), and Yangshin becomes space, embodying the principles of emptiness and existence and the interdependence of form and emptiness. This practice, when done for three years, is referred to in Seon Do as "three years of constant development" (三年乳抱).

In the context of macro-level Kundalini Yoga, this stage corresponds to an advanced practice that is not typically found in classical Indian yoga texts, but rather in the highest stages of Tibetan Vajrayana (Tantric) practice, particularly in Phowa (transference of consciousness). Phowa involves the transference of consciousness, a concept briefly mentioned in Tibetan esoteric practices and closely associated with the highest levels of spiritual attainment.

A notable story related to this process involves Bodhidharma, the Buddhist monk (5-6th century CE) credited with bringing Zen Buddhism to China. His journey and experience of enlightenment are said to have involved such practices of shifting consciousness.

The story of Bodhidharma's encounter with a giant, rotting snake on his journey illustrates a profound level of spiritual practice. According to the story, Bodhidharma saw this huge snake by the side of the road, too big for a person to move, and there were no villages nearby to call for help. To dispose of the snake, Bodhidharma temporarily abandoned his own body and entered the body of the snake, took it to the East Sea, and then returned to find his own body gone. This anecdote, whether historically true or not, symbolizes the advanced stage of practice that Bodhidharma had reached upon entering China.

The next stage of Bodhidharma's journey, regardless of the historical accuracy of the story, is often symbolically represented as the process of facing the wall for nine years (九年面壁). This stage corresponds to the practice of "Yeonheo Hapdo" (煉虛合道), which involves Refining Emptiness and Harmonizing with the Dao (Way). This advanced stage of practice reflects a deepening of the spiritual discipline, where the practitioner engages in deep meditation and inner reflection, symbolized by facing a wall for an extended period.

In Seon Do, this phase of cultivation involves nurturing the newly born spiritual body for three years, a process similar to feeding a newborn baby. When one initiates the emergence of the spiritual body, it requires careful attention each time. When the spiritual body leaves and does not return, it is often due to a lack of depth in the practice and a hasty effort to project it outward prematurely.

The method of projecting the Yangshin (spiritual body) is to enter into a state of stillness and emptiness when the spiritual body is in the upper dantian. First, a pure silver light is projected from the crown of the head, and then, with a single thought, the light follows out of the body. When leaving the body, it is important to return quickly, guided by the white, silver light emanating from within. Once one returns, one must enter into meditation again.

However, it is important to understand that this description is more symbolic than literal. The challenge lies in the illusory space of visions connected to the world of intermediate spirits. The real practice is not about physically traveling somewhere, but about exploring these realms inwardly. Developing the ability to navigate these inner spaces is the essence of cultivating spiritual body, called Yupo (乳哺; development). It is about developing the ability to journey within oneself and expanding inner awareness and spiritual depth.

Returning to Seon Do perspective, Yupo (乳哺; development) refers to the process of nurturing an immature body into a mature entity that embodies the principle of "JinKongMyoYu" (眞空妙有; emptiness of inherent existence). This is the practice of letting the spiritual body return to emptiness. The guiding light for entering and exiting the Yangshin (spiritual body) is the purple-golden light, a light that does not exist in this world and signifies a different dimensional realm. In other words, it means entering another dimension.

The guideline suggests not allowing the spiritual body to come in and out at any time, but to start doing it once every seven days, gradually increasing the distance from near to far. In the beginning, it is important to practice on clear, calm days without wind or lightning. After three months, you can go out three times a day; after six months, five times a day; and after one year, seven times a day. After two years, you can do it regardless of day or night, and after three years, you can travel through heaven and earth without restriction and manifest in countless forms.

This stage transcends the concept of physical space as distance. It signifies an inward journey into one's inner self. The practice reflects a deep exploration of one's inner dimensions and spiritual realms, far beyond the physical limitations of space and time.

After completing Yupo Gong (乳哺功): (the practice of developing and nourishing the spiritual body), then the practice of moving the spiritual body in and out should cease. Instead, one should focus solely on entering deep meditative states of absolute tranquility. Samadhi[41] of total extinction or cessation of perception and feeling (滅盡定), which represents the pinnacle of mindfulness in meditation, then becomes a period of rest and rejuvenation for the spiritual body.

So what happens to the Yangshin (養神; spiritual body)? Does it simply disappear? The answer is no. The Yangshin enters the realm of illusory space-time and merges with the original mind. In cases where this fusion does not occur, the Yangshin can be directed to a specialized study that focuses exclusively on cultivating the spiritual body. This Yangshin study, which transcends the earthly realm, exists in an alternate-dimensional space. It is important to understand that this is not a matter of crossing vast physical distances or engaging in space travel. Rather, it is a journey within oneself, traversing different dimensions of consciousness.

After completing the prescribed training in this particular realm, it is common for the Yangshin (養神: spiritual body) to merge with the Wonshin (元神: original spirit) in the illusory space-time realm known as Saekgye (色界: realm of form[42]). However, there are

---

[41] Samadhi (三昧): Entering a meditative state by letting go of worldly attachments and desires. (死心入定). See page 17.

[42] The "Form Realm" (Sanskrit: Rupadhatu; Chinese: 色界), in Buddhist cosmology, is one of the three realms of existence. This realm is characterized by the presence of

instances where the Yangshin is not projected outward, especially when preparing for the next phase of practice, facing wall meditation (面壁功夫). In some cases, practitioners enter directly into the meditation of absolute tranquility without sending out the Yangshin. This is a path typically reserved for those born with immense spiritual gifts, often predestined to become Cheonseon (天仙; heavenly immortals), Geumseon (金仙; golden immortals), or, in Buddhist terms, high-level bodhisattvas or buddhas.

Up until now, the practice has been about observing the light, whether it is moving within oneself, from within to without, or entering from without. But this next level transcends the physical body. In other words, the consciousness of the physical body disappears, and the practice involves perceiving light, where the universe becomes one's body, and one's body merges with the vastness of space. So, if the previous stages could be compared to Microcosmic Orbit, this stage represents Macrocosmic Orbit. The guidance of an experienced practitioner is highly recommended when studying this process.

D. Cultivating Emptiness and Harmonizing with the Dao (還虛合道)

The nine year facing the wall meditation, which corresponds to the Samnyeon Yupo[43] (三年乳抱, three year practice), involves a process in which, after thoroughly maturing the Yangshin (養神: spiritual

---

form and subtler degrees of sensations as compared to the Desire Realm (Kamadhatu), which is dominated by the coarser sensations and desires.

[43] Three years of constant practice while in seclusion and dedicated to deep meditation and spiritual cultivation.

body) and understanding the principles of heaven and earth, the practitioner no longer sends the Yangshin out separately. Instead, the training now focuses on spreading the form of the Yangshin throughout the universe, essentially transforming it into Emptiness. To accomplish this, it is crucial to no longer separate the Yangshin from the physical body and send it out.

At the same time, the practitioner's physical body goes through a process of merging with the Emptiness, following the Yangshin. This practice is known as Hugong Bunsae (虛空粉碎; Shattering the Void [44]) or Manghyeong (忘形; forgetting form). This transformation is boundless and is considered the most difficult stage. It is a level of practice beyond the reach of ordinary practitioners. Here, the concept of 'self' ceases to exist, leading to a state of true emptiness and wonderful existence (眞空妙有), where one is neither existent nor non-existent.

When a person completely forgets the physical body, the Yangshin becomes one with the great Void/Emptiness, a process called Yeonheo (煉虛; refining emptiness). This stage of practice doesn't have a definite endpoint. Achieving the complete dissolution of the physical body into emptiness, or Hugong Bunsae (虛空粉碎; Shattering the Void), naturally means reaching the stage of Yedo Hapjin (與道合眞; Unification with the Dao), where one becomes one with the Dao.

There is a form of training that is different from the process of dissolving the body into the Void, in which one retains one's physical

---

[44] Hugong Bunsae: the process of dissolving one's physical body and merging it with the universe or the void through deep meditation and spiritual cultivation

form but makes it so that no shadow is cast. This approach is relevant to the stage of Yeon-Jeong-Hwa-Qi (煉精化氣; refining essence into energy), where the practitioner continues to transform the material components of the body into Qi without moving on to the next stage of creating small elixir and advancing to the stage of Yeon-Qi-Hwa-Shin (鍊氣化神; refining energy into spirit) for the creation of great elixir. What happens then? Since the material aspect of the body is essentially made up of the essence of the grains, that essence is transformed into Qi, just like in the process of refining Qi. As a result, even though the physical form remains, the body is composed of Qi, which allows light to pass through it. This leaves only a very faint shadow, which is practically nonexistent. This phenomenon is common among Tibetan meditators who practice Tummo (Inner Heat) in remote mountain caves, where they continuously generate vital heat without much contact with the outside world.

The ultimate stage of practice is to harmonize with the natural order of heaven and earth, to transcend the earth and wander freely through the galaxy, embodying the realm of the divine as described in Zhuangzi's chapter on "Free and Easy Wandering"[45] (逍遙遊). This state represents the pursuit of ultimate freedom, a liberation that can only be achieved when one completely disappears from the constraints of time and space. The goal is not only to achieve a state of Mindlessness (無心, Mushim), but also to achieve Formlessness (無形). This path can only be reached through the practice of Effortless

---

[45] Zhuang Zi's chapter on "Free and Easy Wandering" from the book named for the author, Zhuang Zi (4th century BCE, China).

Action[46] (無爲, Wu Wei), which has always been considered the highest and ultimate stage of cultivation. Remembering that all our efforts ultimately reside in the realm of Yu Wei (有爲 [47]), which is bound by birth and cessation, is important. Birth and cessation are cyclic in nature, a cycle that encompasses all phenomena, including ourselves.

Ordinary beings, or Beombu[48] (凡夫), have never experienced anything beyond this cycle and cannot even imagine what lies beyond it. No matter what they imagine, their minds are inevitably caught up in this endless cycle of birth and death.

---

[46] Wu Wei: "Non-Doing" or "Effortless Action." Is a fundamental Daoist principle that suggests the best way to live is in natural accord with the flow of life, without force or excessive effort.

[47] Yu Wei: "Having Action" or "Active." It is often used to describe actions that are deliberate, contrived, or forceful, as opposed to the natural and spontaneous action.

[48] Beombu: "Ordinary Person" or "Common Man." It refers to people who are not enlightened or spiritually cultivated, who are caught up in the mundane and material aspects of life.

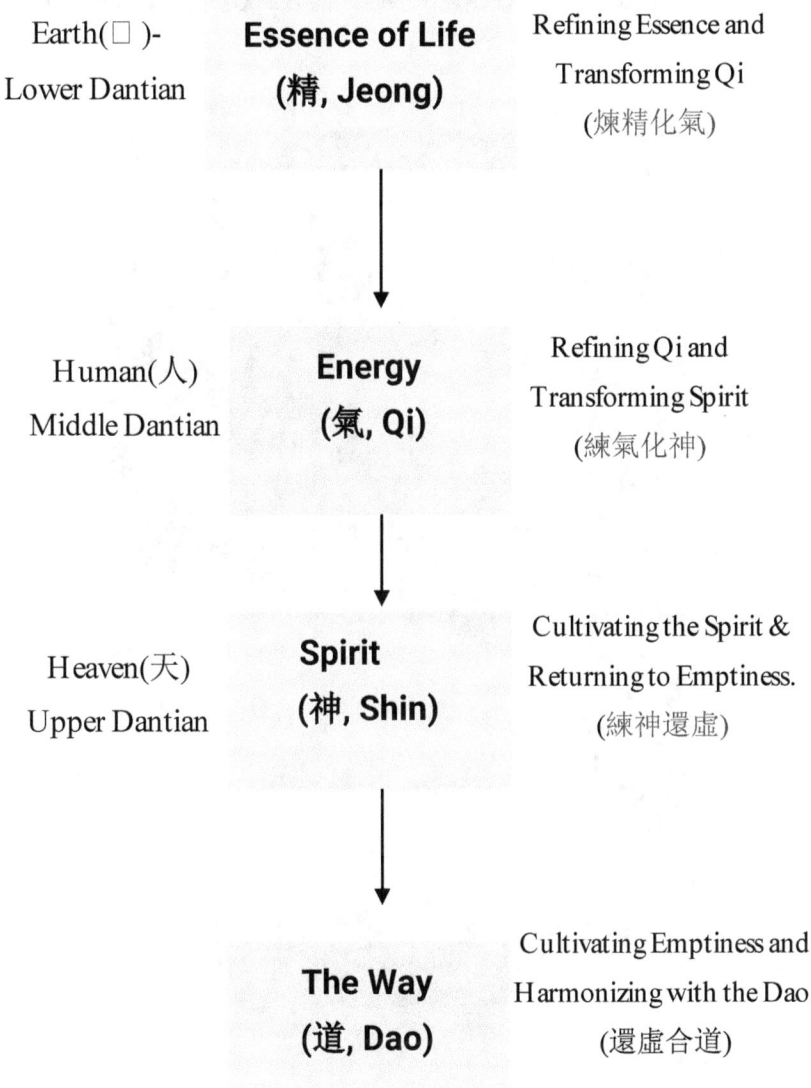

Chapter IV. Seon Do: Way of Immortals

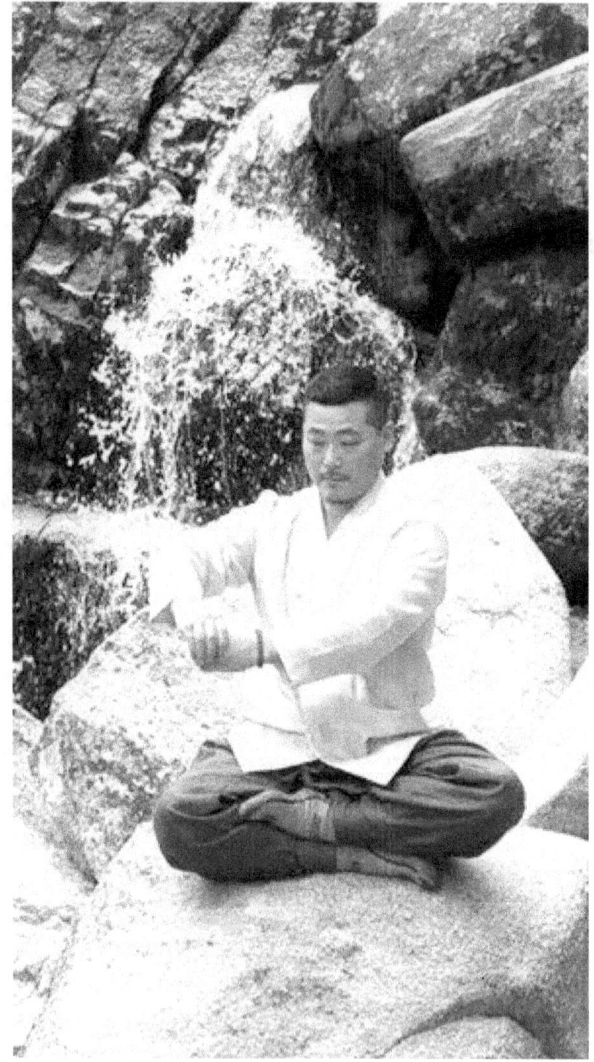

Master Sang Han in Meditation

A. What is Seon Do?
Why Should Humans Practice Seon Do?

Seon Do (仙道), or the "Way of the Immortal," is the path by which humans evolve and become free from all the misery, bumps and bruises of current human limitations. Historically, those who transcended the typical human condition were known as "Seon." They chose a path of an interior life up in the mountains versus staying in the more common cities and villages. This was a conscious decision to abandon the conventional human lifestyle of forming communities, marrying, procreating, and inevitably succumbing to illness and death, all within a competitive framework of survival. Social norms, or the cycle of life and death, did not bind Seon individuals.

The concept of a "Seon" person was not unique to Korea or China, but was a common development in civilizations such as India, the Middle East, and Egypt, which eventually contributed to the birth of the various religions practices.

Among the diverse spectrum of global spiritual traditions, practices like Seon Do and Yoga stand out for emphasizing practical spiritual cultivation. Known for their profound influence on various spiritual paths, these traditions have successfully maintained their unique identities. This is largely due to their focus on comprehensive, experiential practice, which allows practitioners to engage with spirituality beyond the confines of specific doctrines. As a result, Seon Do offers paths that focus on personal spiritual development and resonate with those seeking a direct and experiential approach to understanding and living spiritually through mind/body connection.

As for why these beneficial paths like Seon Do aren't more widely practiced, it is important to consider their historical context and accessibility. While these paths have proven effective, their teachings have traditionally been kept mysterious, perhaps due to the prevailing levels of societal consciousness in the past. In earlier times, social structures often emphasized the consolidation of power among a few, with less emphasis on individual autonomy. This environment led to the marginalization of many reformers and spiritual seekers. In today's liberal societies there is a greater appreciation for individual dignity and freedom, creating an environment in which diverse spiritual paths can be openly explored and discussed. This shift reflects a growing recognition of personal choice in lifestyle and spiritual practice, allowing for a broader exploration of different spiritual paths.

From a quantum theory perspective, humanity is interconnected and functions as a single organism. As individuals evolve, that evolution affects the entire species. The evolution of each individual contributes to the collective evolutional whole of humanity.

This interconnectedness means that each individual's progress isn't isolated but is part of the evolution of the entire species. Like cells in a body, enlightened individuals could be considered the brain cells of humanity, storing untapped potential. Going forward, humanity must develop a closer, more organic interconnectedness to progress. This interconnectedness is essential for awakening the our dormant capabilities within the human brain.

Seon Do is about transcending human limitations, achieving harmony with nature, and freeing oneself from worldly suffering. It is a path that emphasizes practical spiritual cultivation, leading to the evolution not only of the individual but of humanity as a whole. Through such practice, individuals can tap into their spiritual potential and contribute to the collective evolution and betterment of humanity.

To clarify the difference between Qigong, Yoga, relaxation techniques, and conventional low-impact exercises, Qigong practice consists primarily of internal energy activating and developing exercises, breathing exercises, meditation, stretching, and physical movements all pursued with a heightened sense of feeling, focus and awareness of the subtle energy of Qi. This is what differentiates Qigong. This state of being present with the Qi, in turn, plays a key role in healing and health.

B. Overview of Sojucheon and Kundalini

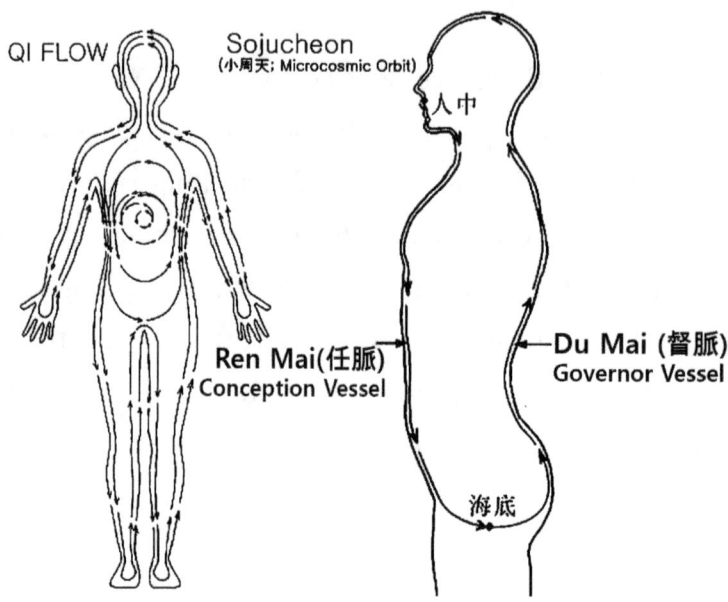

In the practice of Sojucheon (小周天; Microcosmic Orbit) there are various specific actions. The first is Zha Wu Jucheon (子午周天; Conception and Governor Vessel Circulation), which circulates energy along the Ren Mai (任脈; Conception Vessel) and the Du Mai (督脈; Governor Vessel). The second is Kan Li Jucheon (坎離周天; Circulation of Heart and Kidney Qi), which circulates energy between the heart and kidneys. The third is Geongon Jucheon (乾坤周天; a path of circulation which starts from Baeghoe (百會; GV20) at the crown of the head moving throughout the body, reaching Yongquan (涌泉; Kidney 1) on the sole of the foot; this path involves circulation through the Eight Extraordinary Vessels (奇經八脈), which encompasses the entire body.

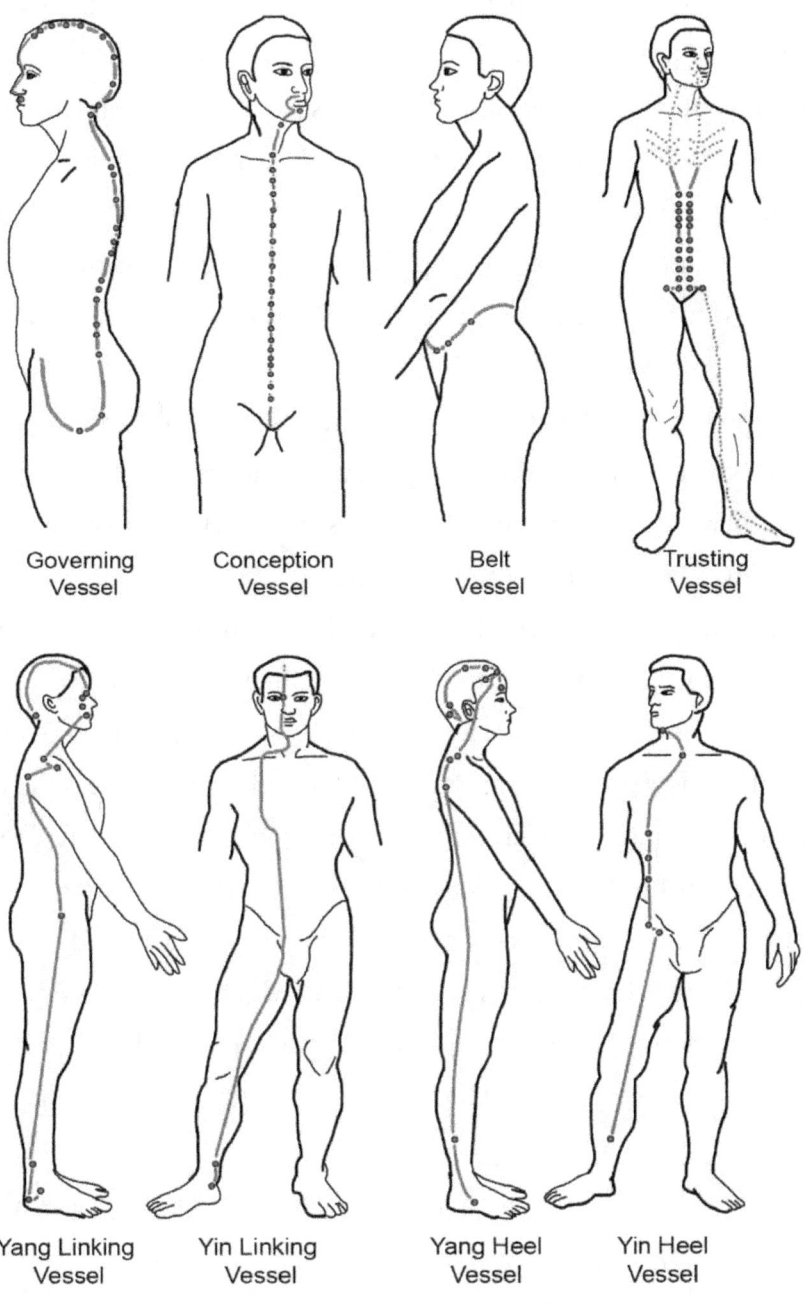

Eight Extraordinary Vessels

Similar to Seon Do, where the practices are divided into Sojucheon (小周天; Microcosmic Orbit) and Daejucheon (大周天; Macrocosmic Orbit), Kundalini in yoga also has two aspects: Micro Kundalini and Macro Kundalini. The practice of Hatha Yoga, known for its focus on asanas (postures), is primarily aimed at awakening the Micro Kundalini as a preparatory step. In Seon Do, this corresponds to practices such as Qigong exercises (氣功體操) and Qi Leading Techniques[49] (導引術).

In the practice of Kundalini Yoga, the first concept encountered is 'Nadi', which means 'channel' or 'pathway'. Nadi refer to the channels through which 'Qi', or bioenergy, flows, and includes electrical and magnetic forces[50]. Nadis can be likened to the nerve endings of the autonomic nervous system that are distributed throughout the human body. According to Tantric scriptures, there are 72,000 Nadis or energy channels in the human body; fourteen are considered the most important. The three central Nadis are Ida, which carries the energy of water, beginning at the left nostril and running down the left side of the spine to the tailbone; Pingala, which carries the energy of fire, beginning at the right nostril and following a similar path down the right side of the spine; and Sushumna, which is associated with electrical energy. Nadis are important neural circuits within the body that are integral to its energetic framework. In the context of chakras,

---

[49] Qi Leading Techniques: The stretching techniques that guide and lead Qi (energy) throughout the body.

[50] Qi is bio energy in different subtle energy forms, such as electric, magnetic, and far-infrared radiation. These forms of subtle energy function through an energetic network in the body for coherent communication between all the body's organs, tissues and cells; between the mind and body; as well as between body and the living environment.

or energy centers, the Nadis: Ida, Pingala, and Sushumna intersect about three times, forming knots.

From a medical perspective, this concept can be understood in terms of the sympathetic and parasympathetic nervous systems. The sympathetic nervous system, corresponding to the Pingala Nadi, associated with fire energy, works in harmony and balance with the parasympathetic nervous system. When this balance is disturbed, it can lead to a weakened immune system and a predisposition to allergic conditions such as rhinitis. Rhinitis typically manifests as a blockage in one nostril; if the left nostril is frequently blocked, it indicates an excess of internal heat. This is because the right nostril, and therefore the Pingala Nadi, becomes overly active, resulting in weakening of the parasympathetic nervous system compared to the activity of the sympathetic nervous system. This imbalance can make individuals more susceptible to circulatory disorders.

Conversely, if the right nostril is predominantly blocked, the left nostril and consequently the parasympathetic nervous system, will be overactive. This condition can lead to a sluggish metabolism, making the individual more susceptible to digestive disorders and depression. If left untreated over a long period of time, blockages in one nostril can sometimes cause changes in one's physical constitution or personality traits, even if they were initially caused by physical trauma.

The pathways of Ida, Pingala, and Sushumna are three crucial channels consisting of the central nerve, which runs through the center of the spine, along with the nerves on its left and right sides, which surround the central nerve like two snakes. It is reminiscent of the staff of Hermes in Greek mythology. External Qi (prana[51]) entering the body is distributed through these three primary nerves and their numerous subsidiary channels. The External Qi/prana is then transported and stored in various sensory nerve centers before being distributed to different organs and areas of the body.

When the Ida and Pingala are well balanced, their electrical energy is generated at the energy centers. Such energy is significantly stronger than the bioelectricity produced within cells by cellular respiration. The experience of this potent electrical energy is unique to practitioners of Seon Do and Kundalini, and it is not typically encountered by the general population. In contrast, those who do not engage in such practices tend to perceive life through a binary lens, lacking multidimensional insight, and thus often reduce their understanding of life to a simplistic black-and-white view.

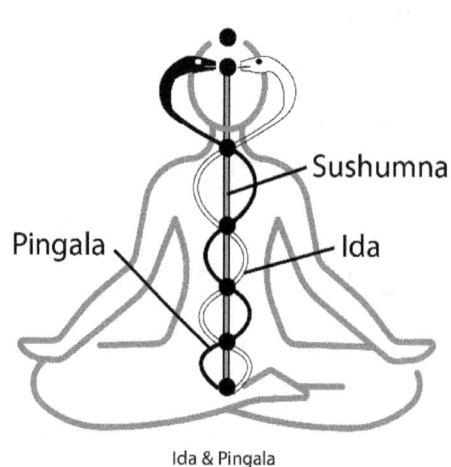
Ida & Pingala

Intensely generated electrical energy flows directly into the Sushumna, the central channel in the middle of the spine. It is when this bioelectricity flows through the Sushumna that the true awakening of Kundalini begins. As a result, dormant regions of the brain awaken,

---

[51] Prana: Vital energy that exists in all things. can include psychic energy.

giving rise to various visions and heightened sensory experiences. This awakening leads to a dimensional categorization of life, transforming one's understanding into a more multifaceted perspective.

C. About the Energy Centers

In the realm of Sojucheon, we can make comparisons to Kundalini practice. Let us cross over to a look at the Kundalini Yoga viewpoint in this section. Certain central energy centers are integral to its understanding and execution. These energy centers are known in yoga as chakras, a Sanskrit term that translates to "Wheel." This name comes from their characteristic behavior, where the energy at these points appears to swirl in a pattern similar to a vortex, evoking the image of a spinning wheel. These energy centers, or chakras, can be compared to "vortices" in modern terms.

It is widely accepted in various spiritual and scientific studies that energy throughout the universe tends to manifest in these vortex formations, a concept visibly demonstrated in the movement of water. Similarly, our human body is host to these dynamic energy vortices, the chakras. Their presence and function within us have been confirmed by numerous studies and traditional practices, highlighting their crucial role in both Kundalini Yoga and the broader understanding of our body's energy dynamics.

1. Coccygeal Plexus : Seminal Vesicle-Males/Womb-Females

In Sanskrit, this first energy center is known as the Muladhara chakra. Muladhara" translates to "root," indicating its foundational role. In the context of Seon Do, it corresponds to the Hoeeum (CV1; perineum) acupressure point, but more specifically, it refers to the lower Dantian energy point. Therefore, it is located near the testicles for men and near the uterus for women. A snake coiled three and a half times symbolizes the dormant Kundalini energy, representing this energy center. When this center is stimulated through conscious breathing techniques, it begins to awaken the Kundalini energy, initiating the process of spiritual awakening.

Once the energy center is awakened, the dormant serpent symbolizing the Kundalini energy begins to stir, eventually lifting its head. This process involves the serpent moving from the base of the spine, through the tailbone, up along the spinal column, to the brain. This journey, in the context of Seon Do, is referred to as the Microcosmic Orbit, with the highest dimension of this process aligning with the path of Dan Do (丹道; the Way of the Elixir). The image of a cobra raising its head and moving up through the spine in Kundalini practice is analogous to the depiction in Seon Do of a dragon ascending while grasping a pearl.

In certain yoga texts, there is a description of what happens after the initial awakening of the kundalini energy. The process involves the energy, symbolized as a snake in the brain, descending through the energy pathways to settle in the chest. This experience is believed to bring about a profound realization of one's True Self.

A parallel concept in Seon Do is a stage known as O Ryong Bong Seong (五龍奉聖; involving the guidance of five dragons directing the elixirs to the middle Dantian). In this stage, five dragons engage and move the energy, or elixir, known as dan to the middle Dantian, thereby opening a significant spiritual ground. This is part of a larger process that includes passing through the Great Elixir stage, where the elixir (Dan) resides and harmonizes in the middle Dantian, eventually converging with the original spirit. This convergence results in the transformation and eventual separation of the spiritual body (Yang Shin), marking the height in one's spiritual journey.

In the Macro Kundalini stage, the focus of practice shifts from the physical body to a more spiritual and mental discipline. This phase triggers numerous awakenings and transformations of consciousness, progressively aligning the practitioner with a more universal and divine existence. At this point, the practitioner transcends the limitations typically associated with human beings on Earth. They become cosmic beings, existing on a spiritual plane akin to that of a deity, transcending ordinary human experiences and limitations. This evolution marks a significant shift from a purely physical or earthly perspective to a broader, more expansive universal consciousness.

The appearance of a golden pearl[52] within the Muladhara root energy center indicates the awakening of this center, signaling the beginning of a profound spiritual awakening. Initially, visible light may not accompany this awakening, but it may be felt as electrical stimulation or sensations of heat and cold. The appearance of the pearl signifies the advanced stage of the process in which the water and fire elements combine to generate electricity, known as the phase of refining essence into energy. At this stage, the brain ceases to dissipate electrical energy into random thoughts and instead begins to collect and transform this energy into light.

---

[52] Golden Pearl is also called Golden Pill

At first, the light in the energy center may appear faint and blurry, resembling a tiny white grain, but as the Sushumna (central energy channel) is passed through repeatedly, the interaction of the fire and water energies of the body are transformed into electric energy, which accumulates and increases in intensity. When the light reaches the size of a pearl, it transforms into a radiant golden color. At this point, one may experience sudden flashes of light in front of the eyes or electric shocks along the spine that cause shaking or frequent dreams of snakes. There may also be sensations of hot or cool currents or the feeling of a stream of water running up the spine and across the body as if a river runs through the abdomen.

Experiences vary from person to person and are common precursors to an inevitable stage in the spiritual journey. Such sensations can evoke a deep sense of the unknown that can be unsettling. This can lead to a sudden fear of death or, conversely, a release from the fear of dying. Abrupt and unpredictable changes can throw a practitioner into confusion as the surface consciousness struggles to make sense of changes. These are signs that the subconscious is beginning to awaken, shifting the weight of consciousness from the surface to the deep unconscious and prompting the practitioner to prepare for an impending transformation.

In truth, when people are said to "lose their minds," it is only the surface consciousness that becomes unhinged; the subconscious cannot go mad. From the perspective of surface consciousness, the subconscious always appears to be in a state of madness. As Kundalini progresses, such phenomena can become more bizarre and intense.

With time, the practitioner develops resilience, becoming less startled by these experiences, but initially, one's entrenched beliefs can lead to mental turmoil.

In addition, it is important to note that the golden light within the energy center may sometimes emit a reddish, flaming hue. This occurrence signifies a peak in the vitality of the energy center, representing the transformation of Jeong (essence of life) into Qi.

2. Sacral Plexus (Spermatic Cord, Ovaries)

In Sanskrit, the second energy center is known as the Swadhisthana Chakra. Swadhisthana means the dwelling place of the individual self, or ego. It is located at the coccygeal nerve complex or in the lower abdominal nerve plexus. In terms of hormonal glands, in men, it corresponds to the testes, which are external to the body, and in women, it corresponds to the ovaries; both produce sex hormones. These sex hormones have been a driving force in the advancement of civilization and are considered the most important hormones for humans to date.

While the Muladhara (root) chakra is associated with strong survival instincts, the Swadhisthana chakra is strongly associated with reproductive instincts. The normal consciousness of human beings on Earth resides predominantly in this energy center. The color associated with this chakra is blue, symbolizing its connection to the water elements and the moon, and it has a direct relationship to the water energy of the kidneys.

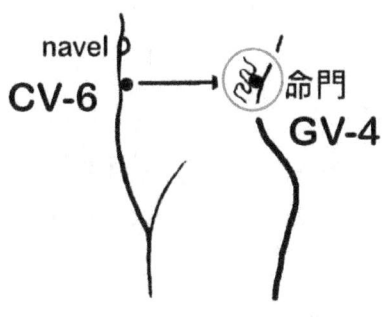

When the Swadhisthana chakra is awakened, or when Kundalini energy resides in this center, a significant increase in sexual sensation and potency is often experienced. When a practitioner no longer feels any sexual ability or desire, it indicates that they have transcended this energy center. At this stage, there is no longer any struggle with or suppression of primal instincts.

In Seon Do, this energy center corresponds to the Myeongmun acupoint point (GV4) in the Du Mai (Governing Vessel) and the Qihai acupoint point (CV6) in the Ren Mai (Conception Vessel). However, because this energy center is fundamentally related to the Zhong Mai (Trusting Vessel)[53], It is located about two-thirds of the way into the body along the Ren Mai (Conception Vessel) and one-third of the way into the Du Mai (Governing Vessel).

3. Solar Plexus (Adrenal Glands)

In Sanskrit, the third energy center is known as the Manipura Chakra. Associated with the element of fire, Manipura is located behind the stomach area and is connected to the adrenal glands on top

---

[53] See page 97.

of the kidneys. It is the site of the secretion of adrenaline, a steroid hormone that plays a crucial role in the body's vitality and energy levels. When activated, the Manipura Chakra often manifests innate talents in martial arts and sports. In addition, strengthening this center can endow an individual with charisma and dignity, attracting numerous followers. This center is connected to what is known as the etheric body, or Crown Chakra GV 20 (魄體, Baeghoe), from which true human nature emerges.

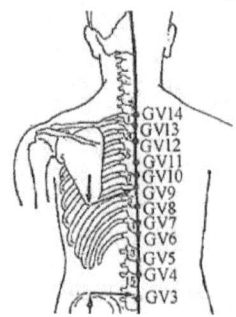

True human nature is the instinct that emerges once we have transcended animal tendencies and marks the very first traits that are exclusively human. It is at this stage of energetic progression that one truly begins to develop an interest in the spiritual realm. This energy center is aptly called "Jewel City." In the practice of Seon Do, this center is associated with the Hyeobcheog Point Governor Vessel (GV6) and the Conception Vessel CV12 (Jungwan Point).

4. Thoracic Plexus (Thymus)

In Sanskrit, the fourth energy center is called the Anahata Chakra. Anahata means immortality and is often associated with the heart. More specifically, it corresponds to the thymus gland, which plays a crucial role in the immune system. When the Anahata Chakra is awakened, one's sensitivity becomes acute. This heightened sensitivity is the basis for empathy, not only with humans, but also with other species. Without this refined sensitivity, a person may find it difficult to connect and empathize with animals, plants, and fellow human beings, including experiencing the emotion of love.

The fourth energy center can be called the middle energy center, which encapsulates the most human aspects. It is at this fourth energy center level that true human nature, humanity, and personality are expressed, resonating and moving all who encounter them. In Golden Rishi Qigong we refer to the middle energy center as the Middle Dantian area.

As this energy center begins to awaken, there is a natural communion with nature. One may feel a strong pull toward wooded forests and seek solitude away from people, finding peace in the quiet of nature. There is often a deep longing for a pastoral, rural life. However, when the Anahata Chakra is fully awakened, it gives rise to a boundless flow of compassion, making the need for a specific place less important. From this point on, the energy known as Shakti, often personified as a goddess, begins to be beautifully represented in Kundalini practice.

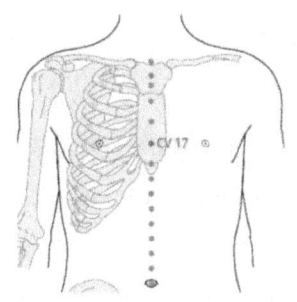

Before reaching this state, the experiences in Kundalini practice can be intense, terrifying, or even bizarre. The Anahata Chakra is where the inner spirit (靈) resides, making it a pivotal point in spiritual practices. In Seon Do, this energy center is particularly referred to as "Spirit Tower" (靈臺, Youngdae) the GV10 point on the Governor

Vessel. On the Conception Vessel, it corresponds to Jeon Zhung (膻中, CV17).

This inner spirit (靈) is analogous to the 'Eighth Consciousness' or 'Alaya-Vijnana' in Buddhism and the 'True Self' in Yoga. As this energy center begins to awaken, individuals may start experiencing a presence during meditation, often accompanied by a sense of profound, serene sadness.

Subtle sadness, known as "Bi-sim" (悲心), reflects the emotional state of the spirit and is one of the deepest human emotions. This sadness, when focused on deeply, leads to a gradual fading of physical consciousness. The awakening of this particular energy center unfolds in six distinct stages:

- First Stage: This stage is marked by the perception of a faint, milky-white ball of light that is somewhat blurred.
- Second Stage: This stage involves an enlightenment regarding the principle of causality—an understanding of the intricate relationship between cause and effect.
- Third Stage: The initial white orb of light gives way to a brilliant crimson orb that greatly enhances the practitioner's emotional sensitivity.
- Fourth Stage: A ball of clear blue light appears. This stage is associated with an increased sense of one's own existence and self-worth.
- Fifth Stage: Characterized by the emergence of a ball of white light tinted with subtle shades of all colors mixed together. It is during this stage that one becomes aware of 'Aroiyasik,' a deeper level of consciousness. It also brings about micro-pain

comparable to the sensation of a sharp needle piercing the heart. This intense experience often causes practitioners to pause or even temporarily withdraw from their spiritual journey. This is a critical point where many practitioners experience a bottleneck in their spiritual growth, often resulting in a temporary halt or slowdown in their progress.

- Sixth Stage: Represents a journey through different levels of consciousness and emotional states. Each contributes to the overall spiritual development of the individual. The concept of 'Granthi', which represents an obstacle in the path of spiritual growth, is traditionally known in yoga as 'Vishnu-granthi'. This obstacle often arises from the inherent human tendency to adhere to traditional and moral orders. Essentially, it is the place where human moral fixations reside. There is also a knot or barrier that forms when the energy from the first energy center attempts to enter the sushumna (central energy channel). This serves as a kind of safety mechanism to prevent Kundalini energy from awakening too easily or indiscriminately in anyone. This phenomenon, in the context of spiritual consciousness within human history, indicates a social necessity where only a few individuals within a group are meant to awaken. In addition, there is a final obstacle, the third knot, or 'Granthi', known as 'Rudra Granthi'. This knot represents the barrier of individual consciousness that separates the self from others. Once this barrier is released, a person can truly understand what happiness is.

In the journey of Kundalini awakening, when the energy begins to rise from the Muladhara (root) Chakra, it does not immediately reach the seventh chakra, Sahasrara. In most cases, the energy does not go beyond the third chakra 'Manipura,' but instead retreats. However, if a practitioner is sincere and dedicated, one can transcend the 'Anahata' (Heart Chakra), where the energy does not regress because they have crossed the second major obstacle. This progress takes them to the sixth chakra, which houses the third 'Granthi'. Before reaching this point, they must pass through the fifth energy center.

5. Throat Plexus (Thyroid)

In Sanskrit, the fifth energy center is called 'Vishuddhi Chakra.' This center is known for its association with the intellect and is a hub for intellectual functions, promoting insightful thinking and contemplation. In addition, the Vishuddhi Chakra plays a crucial role in purifying the body. When Kundalini energy reaches this center, it initiates the purification of the body, the ethereal soul (Hon), and the physical/corporeal soul (Baek). Before the purification process begins, individuals may experience excessive salivation and cold-like symptoms, including discharge from the eyes, nose, and mouth, accompanied by considerable discomfort. Once the purification phase is complete, the body is purified, facilitating visions beyond the physical realm.

As the Vishuddhi chakra awakens, glimpses of past-life memories may appear as fleeting visions, though their meanings remain unclear and manifest only as brief scenes. This fifth center marks the beginning of the higher energy centers that transcend the human realm into the divine. It is at this stage that divine qualities begin to emerge. Anatomically, it corresponds to the location of the thyroid gland. In Seon Do, it aligns with the 'Daechu' GV14 (大椎) point in the Governor Vessel and the 'Cheondol' CV22 (天突) point in the Conception Vessel. If this 'Granthi' (knot) remains unopened, even after reaching the GV14 point, the energy will be diverted to the shoulders and cannot rise any further.

6. Hypothalamus (Pineal Gland)

In Sanskrit, the sixth energy center is known as the 'Ajna Chakra.' In Seon Do it is referred to as 'Cheon-Mog-Hyeol' (天目穴), which means 'Heavenly Eye Point,' the Ajna Chakra is closely associated with the pineal gland and is located near the hypothalamus. The pineal gland is located at the back of the brain, centrally aligned with the back of the ears. When this energy center begins to awaken, one may experience the vision of golden lightning flashes, even with one's eyes closed in total darkness. This is the meeting point of two major Nadis (energy channels): the 'Pingala' (fire energy channel) and the 'Ida' (water energy channel).

When the water and fire elements converge properly, they generate electricity at three specific energy centers, each marked by a knot. These centers are the 'Muladhara' (root), 'Anahata' (heart), and 'Ajna' (third eye) chakras. At these centers, the generation of electricity inevitably leads to the perception of light, which signifies the transformation of "acquired Qi" into "innate Qi." While acquired Qi provides energy to the physical body, innate Qi nourishes the etheric soul and the corporeal soul. Therefore, in Kundalini practice, seeing light often means nourishing and strengthening the etheric and corporeal souls, which is the ultimate goal of this spiritual discipline.

When the 'Ajna' (third eye) energy center awakens, individual consciousness fades away, leading to the dissolution of the ego. This transition imbues practitioners with a sense of profound bliss, often interpreted as an awakening or realization. However, this state of bliss, which is an emotion, does not equate to complete absorption in 'Samadhi' or ultimate enlightenment.

The awakening of the 'Ajna Chakra' also gives rise to a sense of immortality, an awareness that the deep inner self never dies, instilling a sense of the sacred. At this stage, practitioners are no longer prone to wandering or delusions. They may experience various visions and encounters with celestial beings and divine realms, appearing both in dreams and waking life. It is important, however, not to become overly absorbed in these visions and lose sight of progress on the spiritual journey.

The pineal gland, associated with the 'Ajna Chakra,' regulates the secretion of melatonin, a hormone that affects sleep. This can either alleviate insomnia or prevent sleep, giving a degree of freedom from the need for sleep. In Seon Do, this energy center corresponds to the "Yintang" (EX-HN3) point on the Ren meridian and the "Okchim" (GV18) point on the Du meridian. The challenge of penetrating this "Jade Pillow" gate symbolizes the difficulty of this spiritual passage, but intense inner heat can "melt" even this obstacle and reveal a hidden secret. This gate is the last major hurdle before reaching the final energy center, called "Sahasrara" (Crown Chakra).

7. The Entire Cerebrum (大腦)

This energy center is not just another chakra, but the In Sanskrit, the seventh energy center is known as the "Sahasrara Chakra," also called the 'Crown Chakra.' This seventh center, not just an energy center, but ultimate point of convergence between a place of residence for energy, represents the ultimate human energy center and the culmination of the spiritual journey. When energy reaches the Sahasrara, it can feel like many light bulbs are turning on at once. The experiences that follow this activation vary greatly from person to person, with each level of consciousness being different and indescribable in words.

A common experience is the feeling of the individual ego dissolving and merging into a vast ocean of consciousness. At this stage, there is a profound sense of bliss, but it is not that one feels blissful; rather, one becomes the essence of bliss itself.

You might also feel like you are immersed in a sea of light. It is as if hundreds of thousands of searchlights resembling lotus petals burst open in the mind, creating a spectacle similar to fireworks. Once someone has this experience, their entire worldview, including their values and consciousness, is transformed. This change alters their perception of time and space and their ability to distinguish between themselves and others. As a result, abilities in the brain, often referred to as "siddhis" or psychic powers, arise in association with this heightened state of consciousness.

And now another realm opens up, different from the world composed of the sum of our five senses. This new dimension, which can be referred to as the "Bardo" or "in-between state," is where the projection of consciousness becomes as vivid as real physical space. This leads to the ability to control dreams at will and even to influence one's reality through these dreams. Subsequently, during meditation, one can enter the state of 'Sammae' (deep meditative absorption). The longer one lives, the deeper their Sammae becomes, gradually transforming their physical body into a 'vajra' (diamond-like) body. Their bones develop into 'Sarira' (holy relics). It is reminiscent of when the Buddha passed away; although his body was cremated, it barely burned, essentially transforming his entire body into a large Sarira, known as 'True Body Relics'.

Sarira refers to a crystalline structure similar to a diamond that represents the transformation of the essence of life (Jeong) into Qi, which then transforms into spirit. This occurs when the spirit undergoes deep meditative absorption (Sammae), resulting in a metamorphosis of both the spirit and the body. Thus, those who have experienced Sammae several times in their lifetime are said to have more Sarira in their bodies.

When a person's kundalini is fully awakened and reaches the Sahasrara, or crown chakra, he is called a yogic achiever.

When such a person faces death, he enters 'Sammae' (deep meditative absorption) by will and merges with the pure light.

Therefore, for them, death is not an end but a seamless continuation of consciousness. Unlike most people who faint and enter an unconscious state at death, a yogic achiever does not experience this separation. Their death is different from that of ordinary people because they do not re-live suffering or unconscious states; they exist only in an awakened state, beyond the reach of sleep or death.

For them, consciousness and sensation merge. In ordinary people, the two are separate, but yogic achievers reside in a unified state of being. This integration means the dissolution of individuality, or ego. For them, death is like a change of clothes; they can consciously choose rebirth. They consciously enter the womb, stay there, and are born with awareness. This process is detailed in the <u>Aham Sutras</u> of the Buddha's teachings, which outline four ways in which beings incarnate:

The first is unconscious throughout conception, gestation, and birth—typical of ordinary beings.

The second is conscious at conception but not during gestation or birth—common among great saints and sages.

The third is consciousness during conception and gestation but not during birth—seen in Buddhas before enlightenment, Pratyekabuddhas, or Bodhisattvas.

The fourth is conscious during all three stages—characteristic of Bodhisattvas on the verge of enlightenment.

If a practitioner's Sahasrara (crown chakra) is awakened in this life as described in the teachings, he will at least be born with the qualities of a saint in his next life. And if they continue to intensify their practice, on the day they reach full accomplishment, they will have the tremendous power to freely traverse all the states of samsara, the cycle of existence, without any interruption in the continuity of consciousness. Thus, they become the conquerors of all material illusions, not slaves to the cycles of life and death but liberators, guides for sentient beings, and a light in the darkness.

In Seon Do, this energy center is called Niwhanhyul (Entire Cerebrum). The path leading to Niwhanhyul through the central channel of the spine is called Hwangdo (Sushumna), which is the path of the seeds of Dan. On either side of this central channel are the channels of Jeokdo (Ida and Pingala), through which Qi (energy) flows. It is said that only when the seeds of dan pass through does the true path of Governor Vessel open. Similarly, in Yoga, the true awakening of Kundalini is said to occur when it rises through the Sushumna Nadi (channel).

D. Sojucheon / Kundalini

Kundalini[54] and Sojucheon are different expressions for the same phenomenon. However, in contemporary Korean Buddhist culture, which plays a central role in the country's spiritual practices, this phenomenon is often perceived as heretical or deviant. In Tibetan Vajrayana Buddhism, this process is called "completion stage yoga" and is considered a highly advanced practice, a necessary step to be taken. In Korea, however, where Zen Buddhism takes precedence, there is a reluctance to disclose the intricate processes leading to enlightenment, as it is seen as contradictory to the nature of Qigong practice.

Nevertheless, even among dedicated practitioners who may not openly discuss the physical changes they experience, many seek to uncover the reasons and mechanisms behind these transformations. So why does this phenomenon occur?

The phenomenon of Kundalini awakening was considered quite rare in the past, not only in India but also in China. It was not something that anyone could easily trigger. As a result, the phenomenon became overly mystified and exaggerated. But that doesn't mean that this phenomenon doesn't happen. A culture arose that revered individuals who experienced this phenomenon as sacred. In yoga, they are called "avatars," essentially embodying the sacred, and in Daoism, they are called "Shenxian," meaning the divine. If one diligently follows the right steps and finds a true teacher, such a

---

[54] Kundalini refers to a concept in Hindu and yogic traditions that represents a form of life force energy or spiritual energy believed to be located at the base of the spine.

phenomenon can indeed manifest. Of course, individual timelines may vary depending on the student's readiness.

The crucial point to note is that in the past, false teachers often exaggerated such experiences, which could lead to misinterpretations or heretical beliefs. However, when it comes to genuine bodily reactions, there is no need to classify them as heresy or deviation. They are physiological reactions, not dogma.

So, what happens when the Kundalini awakens? The first noticeable change is that a person's temperament becomes more meditative. In other words, if someone originally had a dynamic or choleric temperament, it would be transformed into the opposite temperament through the transformation of their Jeong (精; essence of life) into Qi (氣; energy). In the past, this process was called "Refining Essence and Transforming Qi" (煉精化氣). Most of the experiences in contemporary culture that people enjoy today are due to the unimpeded flow of essence without refining it into energy. This flow is directed toward the gratification of the senses, involving the interaction of the five senses (五感)[55] and the six consciousnesses (六識)[56], which contributes to a more complex and pleasurable experience. Therefore, art, literature, and all sensual pleasures tend to satisfy this aspect of human nature. A person whose essence has been transformed into Qi gradually begins to dislike the various cultural phenomena of the world. Such a person eventually turns inward to

---

[55] Five senses: sound, sight, smell, touch, and taste.
[56] Six consciousnesses (六識): In addition to the five sensory consciousnesses, the sixth is the mental consciousness, which includes awareness of thoughts, emotions, and mental processes; the sixth sense is commonly referred to as the intuitive mind or the "mind's eye."

find pleasure and happiness in the process of "Refining Essence and Transforming Qi" (煉精化氣). They are more likely to enjoy the forest and quiet nature because there is something in the dense nature that resonates with the energy changes in their bodies. Such a person naturally abandons worldly desires and noisy urban areas to seek out peaceful natural environments like forests or mountains. We can now call such a person a practitioner because one is more focused on one's own inner being, which is a joyful path.

This transition is not easy because even a practitioner's memory may contain various worldly habits and dissatisfactions. In Buddhism, these concentrated memories of the past are called "micro-afflictions. To reach the state of being able to perceive such subtle disturbances, one must first go through great suffering and reach a sufficient level of tranquility. Only then does one attain the tranquility necessary to perceive these micro-afflictions, like the gentle ripples on the surface of still water.

Up until that point, one's desires may manifest so vividly on the screen of consciousness that it is hard to distinguish between watching an immersive movie and experiencing a dream. The stronger the kundalini energy, the more intense and vivid these inner experiences become. In Seon Do, this phenomenon is attributed to the mindset of over-eagerness ("Sikshin") leading to "Ma (evil)" "Majang" (blocked energy by evil). It is a fight against evil. These obstacles are not external; their origins lie within one's inner being. It is hard to discern whether it is real or imagined.

In the process of Kundalini awakening, these obstacles are divided into three major challenges known as 'Granthi' (knots-doubts). These are encountered in the Muladhara energy center, the Anahata energy center, and finally the Ajna energy center. In Indian terminology, these are called Brahma Granthi, Vishnu Granthi, and Rudra Granthi, respectively. The phenomena associated with each of these stages have been discussed previously.

In any case, when a practitioner successfully overcomes these challenges and reaches the ultimate goal, the Sahasrara[57], they gain the ability to transcend their physical body with their consciousness. From this point on, they essentially begin to study the process known as the Macro Kundalini (大悟達衰), which is called the cultivation of the spiritual body in Seon Do. In Tibetan Buddhism, this process is called "Phowa[58]," which involves the transfer of consciousness out of the body or the ability to travel freely through space. When this process reaches its full potential, one transcends the limitations of time and space, making it the highest level of practice in Tibetan Buddhism.

If we loosely compare the practice of Tibetan Buddhism to that of Seon Do, the practice of Tummo[59] corresponds to Sojucheon and involves generating vital energy through breathing and meditation. In Tibet, where the environment is extremely cold, Tummo practice doesn't focus on circulating cool water in the body to prevent freezing in temperatures below -20 degrees Celsius. Instead, practitioners sit in

---

[57] Sahasrara, often referred to as the "Crown Chakra," is the seventh and highest chakra in the Hindu yogic and tantric traditions.

[58] Phowa, also spelled as "pho-wa" or "powa," is a Tibetan Buddhist practice that focuses on the transference of consciousness at the time of death.

[59] The primary aim of Tummo practice is to harness the body's inner energy, increase the body's temperature, and activate the subtle energy centers (chakras) along the spine. This practice is believed to have both physical and spiritual benefits, including improved health, increased resilience to cold temperatures, and enhanced spiritual insight.

the sun to endure the heat. If their bodies don't produce cool water, they could suffer from heat stroke. But even though it is the same kundalini process, whether to emphasize the water channel (Ida) or the fire channel (Pingala) depends on the practitioner's natural environment. One isn't right, and the other isn't wrong. In Tibet, those who emphasize the fire channel focus primarily on the progress of advancing yang fire (進陽火), where heat rises through the Governor Vessel and the Trusting Vessel to the brain (refer back to the Gikyungpalmaek The Eight Extraordinary Vessels Diagram).

This Tummo practice also represents the refinement of essence into energy (煉精化氣), and the person who excelled at it the most was the saint, Milarepa[60].

After mastering Tummo, the next stage is Clear Light Yoga (淨光明) in Seon Do, which involves the reflection of light. In the Kundalini process, this can be seen as the exchange of light between the astral body in the head and the causal body in the chest. In Zen, this stage is called the Ten-Month Fetus Cultivation and is considered the Refining Qi and Transforming Spirit (鍊氣化神). In Tibetan Buddhism, it is only after reaching this stage that one can practice "Phowa," which is the yoga of the transference of consciousness. This refers to a single body of consciousness known as the intention-born body (意生身), which is the spiritual body and is the next stage of practice after Cultivating the Spirit and Returning to Emptiness (鍊神還虛).

---

[60] Milarepa, also known as Jetsun Milarepa, was a legendary figure in Tibetan Buddhism and one of the most revered and influential spiritual teachers in the history of Tibetan Buddhism.

So what does it mean to transcend the consciousness and cultivate the spiritual body (靈體)? Generally speaking, people don't usually refer to their soul (靈) as their spiritual body. However, those who have experienced the kundalini or sojucheon (microcosmic orbit) for a long time will witness their essence transforming into Qi and then into spirit (神). This transformation eventually provides enough energy for the soul in the mind, which can be called the spiritual body. The spiritual body continues to accumulate divine energy from the head, thereby increasing the power of consciousness. Essentially, it is a process of becoming aware of the presence of the soul. In general, people don't easily perceive the presence of the soul, and this awareness is only achieved through deep practice. This resembles Buddhist practice, where persistent effort allows one to sense the presence of alaya consciousness (alaya-vijñāna) through the micro-afflictions that arise. Alaya consciousness can also be viewed as the activation function of the mental body.

Seon Do doesn't use the terms mental body (靈體) and alaya consciousness (阿賴耶識) but refers to the original spirit. The process of transforming into the original spirit energy is called "Dotai" (道胎) or "Yangtai" (養胎) in Seon Do, also known as the "Daejucheon" (大周天; macrocosmic orbit) process. In yoga, the kundalini process is divided into "small kundalini" (小坤地鱗) and "great kundalini" (大坤地鱗), while in Seon Do it is divided into the "Sojucheon" (microcosmic orbit), the "Dajucheon" (macrocosmic orbit), and the process of cultivating the spirit (養神).

E. Purpose of the Practice

The Sojucheon (Microcosmic Orbit) phenomenon is of immense importance not only in the field of spiritual practice but is also considered necessary in Hinduism, Buddhism, and Daoism. However, undergoing such physical and psychological transformations without caution can pose significant risks. Due to the lack of interest from the general public, these practices have been passed down and refined exclusively within esoteric traditions. For example, yoga represents the esoteric tradition in Hinduism, Tibetan Buddhism in Buddhism, and Seon Do in Daoism.

The question arises: Can we attain the ultimate state through religious teachings alone? While not impossible, even religious practices, upon closer examination, reveal elements rooted in esoteric traditions. Southern Buddhism includes Vipassana Meditation, and Northern Buddhism includes Zen Buddhism. However, as practitioners progress to more advanced stages, physical and psychological changes inevitably occur. This is because human beings are a union of body and mind, and a change in the mind alone can be merely conceptual and therefore weaker.

In essence, true understanding comes only when there is a change in the body. So, what is the ultimate goal of these different systems of practice? Trying to articulate it in words can lead us astray, for goals arise inherently within a particular value system. Values, in turn, are a product of the mind. No matter how noble and metaphysical a value system may be, it ultimately comes from the mind. Practice aims to transcend the mind, but this task is formidable because even the effort to do so comes from the mind.

The topic at hand then, is the practice of cultivating the mind by alternative means, which is often called Sojucheon (Microcosmic Orbit) or the Kundalini phenomenon. This is the use of physical practices to transcend the mind. By bringing about subtle changes in the body through these practices, one has the opportunity to liberate the mind.

In a general sense, it is quite difficult to distinguish the mind from its physical counterpart with ordinary perception. That is because it is a very subtle thing. However, when one goes through the process known as body study, one becomes extremely sensitive to the sensations of the body, which makes it possible to observe the workings of the mind in detail. The functioning of the mind is often compared to the continuous flow of thoughts. Even in attempts to meditate and achieve freedom from all ideas and thoughts, the very effort to do so paradoxically becomes a form of thinking. In essence, it becomes a struggle to be free of all ideas and thoughts, whether it is trying not to have any thoughts or simply observing the arising of thoughts. As a result, the incessant flow of thoughts remains uninterrupted. Our soul, like a breath, is constantly engaged in the exchange of information manifested as the coming and going of thoughts. Interrupting this flow, even for a brief moment, puts our soul into a state of suspension, similar to how our physical body experiences brain death after the cessation of breathing for ten minutes. Our mind and soul undergo hundreds of exchanges of information in the form of thoughts every minute.

So what exactly is "freedom from all ideas and thoughts" (無念無想) It means a special state of being that goes beyond the mere cessation of thinking. It is the moment when perceiving a subject arises without any thought of its perception. This state is characterized by the absence of thought processes, which allows the subject to comprehend everything without the interference of thought. Paradoxically, however, the subject itself remains imperceptible. This state eludes conventional consciousness, which typically conflates thought and mind as one. Moreover, this state resists recognition—even the recognition that "no mind" is just another thought. Imagine catching a glimpse of the state of "no mind" through the clouds of thought, much like the sun's rays breaking through the clouds.

This spiritual enlightenment inherent in a person or being is called "inherent spiritual brightness" (本性靈光). In Zen Buddhism (仙佛敎), it is expressed as conveying the idea that the original and inherent nature of the mind is luminous or possesses a spiritual brightness. This "inherent spiritual brightness" is a state of enlightenment, another aspect of the mind, without any consciousness or discernment between living or death. It transcends all truth and falsehood, good and evil, and beauty and ugliness. In the end, the moment of realization is when all efforts in practice come to rest, so we can consider it our ultimate goal. After realization, there is no longer a need to strive for anything. It transcends all truth and falsehood, all good and evil, all beauty and ugliness. The efforts of the sages are to achieve this realization, but in reality, none of them see the moon that the finger is pointing at. They only see the finger itself. If one has achieved a certain level of cultivation practice in previous lifetimes and entered deep

Samadhi[61] (三昧), one can follow the finger's direction and see the moon. Otherwise, the path of Sojucheon or Kundalini must be taken to reach the goal, because it is the path, the inner journey.

Even if one is in deep Samadhi for a long time, it is not easy to experience a complete state of freedom from all thoughts. This is because Samadhi does not necessarily mean no mind. Therefore, Samadhi is also divided into states of no mind and states of mind. It is said that one attains enlightenment by experiencing the state of no mind samadhi, which is called "Musang Sammae" (無想三昧). It is just another expression of the same state. Gradually climbing the steps of Existential Samadhi (有種三昧) does not lead to achieving this state of no mind. Therefore, it is difficult and rare to achieve enlightenment. Experiencing enlightenment means stopping perception, and it is a state of no mind (無心), so the term does not fit the original state well. Maybe people are often misled because it has the opposite nuance. Maybe it was made that way on purpose. With so many people bragging about their enlightenment, it is necessary to distinguish whether it is real or fake.

Those who truly experience such a state do not need to boast about their experience because they realize that there is nothing to be gained. Many people expect and talk about compassion arising when they reach this state, but in reality, compassion cannot arise there. Compassion is an emotional function that arises from one's value system after experiencing such a state. Of course, such emotional

---

[61] Samadhi: A state of meditative consciousness for the attainment of spiritual liberation, joyful calm, beyond absolute bliss.

functions are not a temporary illusion of consciousness but rather a natural ecosystem arising from fundamental emotions. This Seon Do meditation is designed to ensure the survival of the entire human race. One must lead those who follow it in order to achieve overall evolution. This is also a sense of responsibility, where leaders must lead those who follow.

The ultimate goal of Seon Do (the Way of the Immortals; 仙道) is to attain a state of freedom from all ideas and thoughts. In Seon Do philosophy, it is said that without an empty mind, all efforts are in vain. Therefore, the phrase "Sasim-ipjeong" (死心入定; devotion to meditation to the point of death) is commonly used, meaning that the mind must undergo a form of death for liberation, and this state must be maintained for a certain time, not just a fleeting moment. In the realm of Seon Do, the term "Myeoljinjeong" (滅盡定; the highest state of mindfulness in meditation) is used instead of enlightenment. In contrast, Buddhism often uses the term "enlightenment," what is it really?

It is alternatively expressed as seeing one's true nature, which indicates the recognition of one's inherent nature. This implies the existence of an observer who perceives his or her authentic nature. The crucial moment when the brilliance of one's true nature (本性靈光; innate spiritual brilliance) is revealed corresponds to a complete state of samadhi without form, in which cognitive functions are nonexistent. However, the onset of cognitive function occurs upon exiting this state, resulting in a momentary convergence between the radiance of one's true nature and cognitive function, imprinting a profound memory of this encounter. The intricacies of cognitive function are elucidated with meticulous detail, similar to a person falling off a cliff and suddenly remembering their entire life. This extraordinary phenomenon allows for rapid observation of each stage of cognition. In Buddhism, this is called "ilbyeor" (一瞥; momentary realization). While this description may face translation challenges, words remain the only means to convey this phenomenon.

Is there a process in Seon Do that pursues such a state? The stage called Yeon-heo-hap-do (煉虛合道; Refining Emptiness and Harmonizing with the Dao) refers precisely to this state, where after releasing the Yangshin (養神; spiritual body), the practitioner goes through a process called Samnyeon Yupo (三年乳抱; three year practice). This is known as Yeon-shin-hwan-heo (鍊神還虛, Cultivating the Spirit and Returning to Emptiness), but Yeon-heo-hap-do (練虛合道) corresponds to the very last stage in Seon Do, similar to the nine year wall gazing process and is not a practice. In Buddhism, sitting and facing a wall may be a practice. But in Seon Do, it symbolizes a state which means that someone who has experienced emptiness has turned his mind away from the world.

The process of facing the wall for nine years could be seen as a process of pursuing enlightenment in Buddhism. Buddhism goes straight to the pursuit of enlightenment from the beginning, but in Seon Do one naturally encounters enlightenment after going through all the physical training. In Buddhism, enlightenment can be achieved directly without Samadhi (禪定; meditative absorption) or through Samadhi, and Samadhi itself is not the goal; but in Seon Do, enlightenment is seen as the result of Samadhi, a natural byproduct.

So, when they see someone in Seon Do who is pursuing enlightenment as a goal, they say that it is a futile effort because it can seem like a desire to achieve a certain state of consciousness. If they met someone who said that they would ask him why he wanted to achieve enlightenment. Even in Buddhism, this kind of talk has become a typical process. But in Seon Do, if someone answers like that, the master will say that the beginner is very far from the state of Mu-sim (mindlessness). This is because, from the point of view of Seon Do, an empty mind is not seen as a desire. It would be more honest to say that the beginner suffers because he can't achieve an empty mind.

In any case, Seon Do does not deal with the conceptual aspects of any religion or philosophy. This is because it is considered impossible to bring about a transformation of the self while clinging to pre-existing concepts. The mind is the master of the body, and the body follows the mind. At least when the body is healthy.

Seon Do (仙道) teaches first that the state of body and mind should become one. This process, which focuses mainly on guiding and leading technique (導引術) and movement exercises, is called Dong-gong (動功; Movement Exercise). Body and mind becoming one is a process that is not often discussed in typical Seon Do literature. In fact, this process is largely omitted from virtually all Daoist scriptures (道藏經). It mainly refers to the stages before entering the "Hundred Days of Qi Cultivation", which is synonymous with "Refining Essence and Transforming Qi." This phase focuses mainly on guiding and directing Qi throughout the body, often emphasizing stretching techniques and dynamic exercises such as Daoinsul (導引術; Tai Chi, Eight Brocades) and Qigong movement exercises.

Anyone who wishes to practice Seon Do is expected to have already completed the physical Qigong training necessary to reach the state of unification of body and mind. However, modern people often skip this step and try to go straight to the hundred days of releasing Qi. The subsequent stages are recorded in the Daoist scriptures (道藏經).

Even in Buddhism, some people sit in the Zen Meditation Hall (禪房) right away without considering the state of their bodies. But if they try to go through the process of "Refining the Essence to Transform Qi" (煉精化氣) without first cultivating their bodies, they will harm themselves. In yoga, to enter the Kundalini process, it was necessary to practice hatha yoga for at least ten years to reach the state of body and mind becoming one (心身合一) in a very quiet place. However, modern people who live in polluted and complicated environments try to enter the "Hundred Days of Releasing Qi (百日斥氣)" stage without first training their bodies. This is an act that brings illness upon oneself. Of course, it may be possible for someone in one's twenties who has just finished military service and is full of vitality, or for someone who has specialized in sports since high school and made it a career, to immediately enter the "Hundred Days of Qi Cultivation" phase. In addition, it should be noted that some places teach Upper Dantian Breathing, the process of "Cultivating the Spirit and Returning to Emptiness" (鍊神還虛), directly without going through the stages of "Refining the Essence and Transforming the Qi" (煉精化氣), or "Refining the Qi and Transforming the Spirit." This is a very dangerous idea. The process of "Refining the Mind and Returning to Emptiness" must be done sequentially after going through the stages of "Refining the Essence and Transforming the Qi" or "Refining the Qi and Transforming the Spirit. Performing upper Dantian breathing without this preparation is likely to drive a person insane or unable to live a normal life. From the point of view of a Seon Do practitioner, this is an unacceptable practice. Anyone who teaches such practices cannot be considered a Seon Do practitioner. It is no different from the Chinese Daoists of the past, who sold pills made of gold and mercury, claiming they were elixirs, and profited from them. No matter how groundbreaking or novel a theory or principle may be, the human body remains the same as it has always been and may even become weaker.

Modern humans have significantly depleted their emotional and mental energy due to the need to remember excessive amounts of information from an early age, which they attempt to compensate for with high-calorie and nutrient-dense foods, as well as various medical treatments. While one could argue that a longer life expectancy is a sign of better health, it is undeniable that, except for a few athletes who engage in extreme physical training, average physical fitness has declined significantly compared to that of our ancestors.

In the past, even non-soldiers casually walked 12-16 miles a day. Some even walked from Busan to Seoul in one month, which requires at least 16 miles a day. If modern people who are not marathon runners or athletes were asked to walk such distances, they would experience a physical breakdown. In such a state, if one tries lower-level breathing exercises and does not experience any remarkable effects, seeking more mystical effects by practicing higher-level breathing exercises or other spiritual practices will only lead one down a path of mental imbalance. As one's body becomes weaker, his mind is more likely to lose sensibilities. Of course, not all of this nonsensical thinking is false; many statements may be true. However, accepting such statements as truth can be extremely harmful. If you hear the sounds of wandering spirits while lying in bed after a stroke, or if you hear the sounds of other spirits entering your body, this is not Seon Do, but superstition or a desire for miracles.

Seon Do practitioners must work on the unity of body and mind before working on the unity of spirit and human (神人合一). This is the Dao (道) and the truth. Therefore, one should not ruin one's body by falling into flattery, as if by one's own ability, one quickly awakened and experienced true emptiness (無心) and deep meditation (禪定). This is a message that applies to both monastic (僧) and lay (俗) practitioners. It is also important to note that many people try to complete the Sojucheon under the guidance and leadership of others. Please remember that borrowing someone else's energy to open the Sojucheon should not be attempted.

Therefore, Seon Do emphasizes the true seed of Dan (Elixir). This refers to the essence of Yang energy condensed into the essence of life, which creates the true essence of Sojucheon, which is not false energy or madness. The problem is not that the path is blocked, but that there is no vehicle to travel on the path. If there is a vehicle to travel on the path, one will acknowledge the fact that one can break through it and focus one's efforts on creating that vehicle with a sense of ease. This vehicle is the medicine (Elixir; 藥) that Seon Do refers to, and as it circulates through the conception and governing vessels, it will be trained and eventually become the true seed of Dan. Only then will the Sojucheon or Kundalini be attained by passing through the center of the spinal column. Believe this without a doubt.

Chapter V. Principles of the Internal Organs

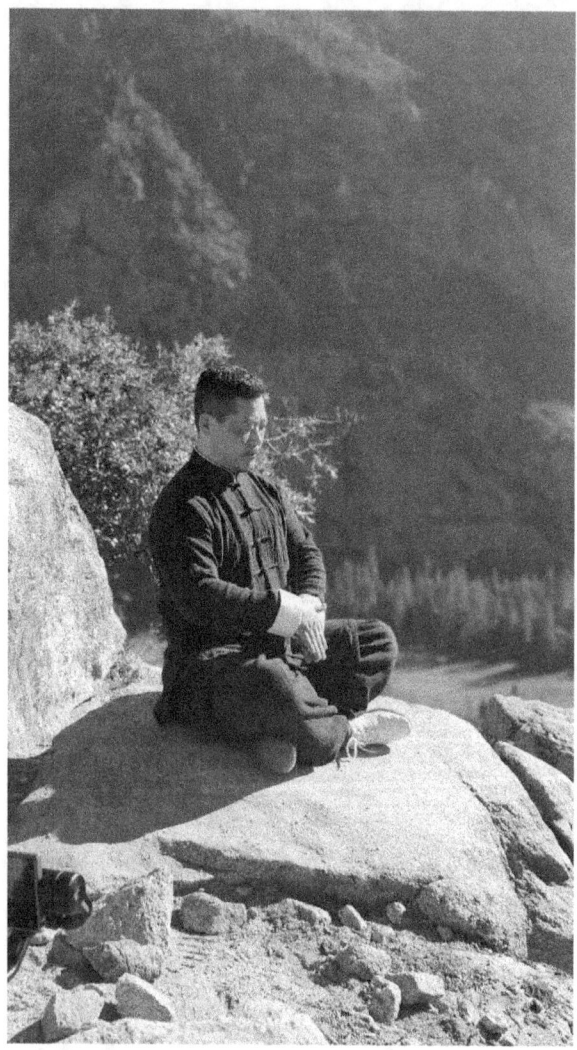

Qigong Energy Massage for Internal Organs

A. The Nature of the Internal Organs

Before delving into the study of Sojucheon, it is important to have a basic understanding of the human body. Sojucheon refers to the circulation of energy produced by the organs in our body. These organs function according to the principles of the five elements and have their own unique order and harmony. Therefore, Sojucheon is essentially the circulation of the microcosm within the body. At its core, circulation is the interplay between the human mind and body, or yang Qi (mind) and yin Qi (body). This is often referred to in Seon Do as the Gamligyogu (坎離交媾; the union of water and fire.) The stages of Gamligyogu (坎離交媾; the union of water and fire) do not belong to the material dimension, it is not the dimension of the essence (精). It is not possible to produce the Great Dan (藥; Elixir) in this circuit. To produce elixir, the circuit must descend to a more material level.

As the circuit becomes more concrete, it moves from the harmony of yin and yang to the harmony of the five elements represented by the elements of fire and water. At this stage, the energy is closer to the essence of life (Jeong) than to Qi, and the fusion of the elements of fire and water creates a medicine (Elixir) that is closer to material quality. This is known in Seon Do as Suhwagije (水火機濟; water and fire reaching harmony.) In yoga, it is said that when the elements of Ida (water, associated with the moon) and Pingala (fire, associated with the sun) are properly blended, the vital energy channel known as Sushumna is activated as the Kundalini, the dormant spiritual energy, is awakened. According to this perspective, there is a circulation between the brain, which controls the fiery energy of the heart, and the lower Dantian area, which controls the watery energy of the kidneys. This circulation is commonly called the Sojucheon, which marks a transition beyond the dimension of mere survival.

When we talk about Seon Do from the perspective of evolution rather than survival, only then does the cultivation method make sense. In the dimension of survival, the tailbone plexus has not yet appeared. The human tail has degenerated, and the potential that is left there has not yet manifested. Therefore, this tailbone needs to be awakened in order to open up the true path of cultivation. In yoga, this tailbone area is called the goddess Shakti, and the relative forebrain is called the god Shiva. When Shiva's messenger awakens Shakti, she ascends the staircase of the spine to unite with the heavenly Shiva, opening the ultimate gate of oneness.

In Seon Do, we are talking about circulation and movement of energy through the lower dantian area, not only a specific acupoint, nor body part, nor single point on the spine. The lower dantian area, a functioning and complex area, is a very important key for the microcosmic orbit. It is another brain-like area. We refer to it as the lower Dantian, which includes the Qihai acupoint (氣海; three finger thickness downward under belly button), the Huiyin acupoint (會陰; perineum), and the Myeongmun acupoint (明門; lower back). The lower dantian cannot be seen anatomically. The upper dantian is where spiritual energy gathers; the lower dantian is where the essence of life is gathered. The spinal cord is the pathway for the water/energy to travel; the entire spinal cord pathway and the cultivated waters moving from the lower dantian to the upper dantian can be called

Suhae (髓海; sea of marrow). But the essence of life (Jeong) has to be cultivated in order to enter the bone to become marrow. When the water/energy enters the bone, it immediately becomes marrow. Therefore, marrow is present in all bones, but the place where it is most abundant is the skull. The special name for the marrow in the skull is the brain (腦). The marrow enters the skull in addition to the essence that enters the tailbone while in the mother's womb. The essence can also enter the bone and change to marrow as it grows. However, in order for the essence to enter the bone, it has to be cultivated, and the necessary process is called Yeon-jeong-hwa-qi (煉精化氣; Refining Essence and Transforming Qi).

However, ordinary people do not experience Yeon-jeong-hwa-qi (煉精化氣; Refining Essence and Transforming Qi) properly. Actually, the flow of Suhae between the cervical plexus and the forebrain is not active, but those who practice Sojucheon in Seon Do or Kundalini in yoga have an active flow of Suhae (髓海). The difference between ordinary people and Buddhas, saints, and immortals lies in the flow of Suhae. Therefore, for those who want to start the path of Seon Do practice by refining their bodies first, awakening this coccygeal plexus is the key to starting the flow of marrow. If the coccygeal plexus is said to correspond to the prostate, testicles, and seminal vesicles in men, it can also be said to correspond to the uterus and ovaries in women. However, rather than designating

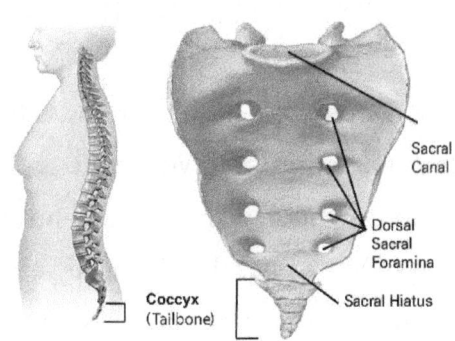

a specific tissue or organ, it can be thought of as a single location. As we discussed earlier, chakras, or energy centers, correspond to organs of the body. These organs can be divided into seven major centers, of which, the second, third, and fourth are associated with our bodily functions. We will now examine the nature of these organs.

The term "Jang" (臟) refers to the internal organ system in the body, while "Sang" (象) refers to the external manifestation of the functions of the organ system. Therefore, the theory of "Jang-sang" (藏象學說) involves the observation of physiological and pathological phenomena outside the living human body to study the activities and relationships of the organ system. This includes all organs, vessels/meridians, and other tissue structures inside and outside the body, as well as their functions, the essence of life, Qi (氣), blood, body fluids (津液), and spirit (神).

In Daoism, the understanding of the physiological functions of the organ system goes beyond simple anatomical knowledge. It is the result of the philosophy of the harmony of heaven and humankind(天人合一), along with Daoist Qigong practice over thousands of years. This understanding was formed through observation and study of one's own living body, verification through experimentation, and the incorporation of the theory of yin-yang and the five elements (陰陽五行) to form a complete theory and doctrine. The main content of "Jang-sang" (藏象學說) theory can be seen from two perspectives: one is to explain the physiological functions, pathological changes, and interrelationships of the organ system, and the other is to explain the physiological functions, pathological changes, and interrelationships of the essence of life (Elixir), Qi, blood, body fluids, and mind, and their relationship with the organ system.

In Jang-sang theory, Jang is not just a simple anatomical concept, but encompasses the concepts of anatomy, physiology, and pathology within the human body system. The physiological function of a Jang includes the physiological functions of several modern organs (臟器), and the physiological function of an organ in anatomy and physiology is related to the physiological functions of several Jangs in Jang-sang theory.

Jangbu (臟腑; organs) is a collective term for the internal organs, which are further divided into the Five Jang (五臟; five organs) and Six Fu (六腑; six bowels) according to their functional characteristics. In addition, there is a non-organ system called the Ki-hang-ji-bu (奇恒之腑.) The Five Jang include the liver, heart, spleen, lung, and kidneys which are each connected to the Six Fu, including the gallbladder, small intestine, stomach, large intestine, bladder, and triple burner. The Jang are considered Yin (陰) and the Fu are considered Yang (陽) in nature, with their corresponding properties following the principle of mutual generation and restraint (相生相剋) of the Five Elements (陰陽五行).

According to Seon Do, an early form of traditional oriental medicine, the Five Jang and Six Fu are not only believed to have unique functions but also to affect one's mental state. The origin of traditional oriental medicine can be found in the Inner Canon of the Yellow Emperor (黃帝內經), where the following passage from the chapter entitled "Essence of Spirit" (本神篇) reads:

"When the heart is excessively agitated, that is, when one is excessively worried and concerned, it damages the spirit. When the spirit is damaged, one becomes anxious, loses oneself, and the muscles and flesh become emaciated; the hair falls out; the complexion becomes dull and dark; and one dies in Winter.

When the spleen is excessively melancholy, that is, when one is lonely and depressed and cannot let go of his emotions, it damages the will. When the will is damaged, the chest gets congested, one cannot move the limbs, the hair falls out, the complexion becomes dull and dark, and one dies in Spring.

When the liver is excessively anxious, that is, when one is afraid or frightened, and the internal organs are excited, the soul is damaged. When the soul is damaged, a person goes crazy, loses one's mind, and cannot behave properly. Such a person's reproductive organs shrink, the muscles contract, one cannot use one's limbs, the hair falls out, the complexion becomes dull and dark, and one dies in the Fall.

When the lungs are too happy, that is, when one has too much joy, it damages your Corporeal Soul (魄). If your vital energy is damaged, you will go mad, and others will not be able to see you. The skin becomes rough, the hair falls out, the complexion becomes dull and dark, and one dies in the Summer.

When the kidneys are overly angry—that is, when one gets angry and can't calm down—it damages the will. When the will is damaged, one forgets what one said before. One cannot bend, stand up, or straighten one's waist and spine; the hair falls out; the complexion becomes dull and dark; and one dies in the last month of Summer."

In this way, each of the five organs (五臟) represents the actions of the five spirits (五神) of Seon Do: spirit (heart, fire, 神), intent (spleen, earth, 意), ethereal soul (liver, wood, 魂), vitality-corporeal soul (lung, metal, 魄), and will-wisdom (kidneys, water, 志), and their excessive activity can cause certain symptoms in the mind and body. The five emotional functions (五情) of these five organs were seen as anger (怒), joy (喜), thinking (思), worry (憂), and fear (恐), to which sadness (悲) and surprise (驚) were added to form the seven emotions (七情). However, this perspective is specific to traditional oriental medicine and may differ slightly from the perspective of Seon Do's Five Elements - Six Emotions (五行六情), depending on one's point of view. In Oriental medicine, excessive emotional activity, especially in joy and anger, as well as fear and surprise, can cause significant illness in the body. The Inner Canon of the Yellow Emperor says, "Madness, shouting, laughing for no reason, and singing are serious diseases caused by great fear." It also says, "Excessive eating, seeing ghosts, and laughing alone in places where others cannot see are diseases caused by excessive joy." Thus, Seon Do and Oriental medicine believe that the body and mind are not separate entities. While Western medicine considers the mind to be the sole function of the brain, in Seon Do, the brain is depicted as a terminal that represents the emotional activity of the five organs and six bowels, called the Sanmyeon (思念, a series of thoughts.) In Seon Do each of the five organs and six bowels of the human body have emotional functions and that they are properly organized in the brain, which is only one part of the non-organ system (奇恒之腑). This way of thinking is similar to quantum theory. Now let's consider the five organs and six bowels in detail.

1. The five organs (五臟)

The five organs have the physiological function of storing and transforming vital energy. They always remain full and do not discharge their contents, so they are always full of vital energy that is acquired but not released. They also contain the essence of mind, blood, and soul. Because they only receive and do not release, they are like the earth, which absorbs without draining. Because they are always full, they have no room for any other substance.

Each of the five organs is associated with a spirit (神) that dwells in it and controls its functions. These spirits are said to show different degrees of activity depending on the balance between positive and negative forces, which are known as morality (性) and emotions (情) respectively. In other words, innate nature (性) and emotions (情) form a pair of complementary forces that correspond to the yin and yang principles of Eastern philosophy.

According to Baekhotong's (白虎通) Morality and Emotions:

"Seong (innate nature) is the active expression of the Yang principle, while essence of life (Jeong) is the passive expression of the Yin principle. Human beings are born from Yin Yang energy, which gives rise to the internal Five Natures and the Six Emotions. This means that the five organs are not just organs that perform physical functions, but are centers where our emotions and mental states flow in and out, and where emotions and mental activity are expressed and regulated. This emphasizes that our emotions are intimately connected to our body's organs and that our physical health and mental state interact. Innate nature is character and emotions, encompassing human nature, temperament, and feelings. The five organs and the six bowels are where 'innate nature' circulates."

In Soh Kil's Theory of the Five Elements, the section entitled "On the Correspondence of the Bowels" outlines the following principles: The Five Elements represent the nature (性) of human beings, while the Six Criteria (六律) embody the emotions (情) of human beings. The nature (性) includes humanity (仁), righteousness (義), propriety (禮), wisdom (智), and trust (信), while the emotions (情) include joy (喜怒), sorrow (哀樂), and love (好惡). The five natures (五性) internally govern the five organs (五臟), while the six emotions (六情) externally govern the six bowels (六腑). Proper regulation of the six bowels leads to the Six Rites (六禮). "Six bowels" refers to internal organs or systems in the body, metaphorically representing internal balance and health. The "Six Rites" (六禮) then symbolize external harmony and order in life or society. The idea is that maintaining internal balance (proper regulation of the six bowels) leads to external harmony (the Six Rites). When internal emotions disrupt natural balance, it can lead to external chaos and disorder. Therefore, in this context, "六禮" (Six Rites) represents the harmonious and orderly conduct of life and society, which is achieved through internal balance and regulation.

Imbalance, disorder, and disharmony can occur when emotions overwhelm nature, emphasizing the critical role of nature in maintaining harmony. The distinction between inner nature and outer emotions is crucial. Emotions, considered yin elements, flow inward through the five viscera, while Nature serves as the foundational essence received at birth. Nature governs stability, ensuring a constant state of calm, while emotions drive movement and change as they interact with the external environment.

Human morality and emotions play a significant role, and an excess of either can affect the five organs and the six bowels, resulting in suffering and disease. The virtues of the Five Natures aligned with each of the five organs are explored to understand the intricate relationship between them.

In Soh Kil's <u>Theory of the Five Elements</u>, the section entitled "On the Correspondence of the Organs":

"The spirit of the liver is to be generous and compassionate. But when grief is excessive, the liver is damaged. When the liver is damaged, what the eyes see is ruined.

The spirit of the heart is to refine one's manners and be truthful. But when one's joy and anger are unrestrained and severe, it hurts the heart. When the heart is damaged, nosebleeds and vomiting occur.

The spirit of the Spleen is to be united, to have thick and strong faith. But if you are selfish and indulge in lust, you will hurt the spleen. When the spleen is damaged, it accumulates and cannot be transformed, and it becomes a blockage disease.

The spirit of lungs is righteous, strong, and resolute, but when you wake up with worries, you hurt them. When the lungs are damaged, the voice is lost through coughing.

The spirit of kidneys is wise, discriminating, and cunning. Over-exertion, over-ambitiousness, and over-motivation damage the kidneys. If the kidneys are damaged, it loses its Jeong (essence of life) and shortens its lifespan."

As such, each of the five organs corresponds to one of the five emotions, and excessive emotion leads to illness. Therefore, wisdom to properly manage the interactions of the five organs is essential to protecting their health.

a. Heart (心)

The heart is located in the chest and is surrounded by the pericardium. Its main functions are to control the blood vessels and the mind. The tongue is the associated organ of the heart. Its representation is on the face; and its emotional changes are joyful. Sweat is the fluid associated with the heart. The heart and small intestine are related in surface anatomy.

The states of abundance, decay, emptiness, and fullness of the heart, blood, and vessels are reflected in changes in the complexion. In healthy individuals, the complexion is rosy and shiny due to proper heart function. In contrast, the complexion of those with heart disease is pale and dull. The pulse is associated with the blood vessels of the heart, and when the pulse disappears, it indicates that the heart is weak and exhausted, leading to blood congestion. Blood is originally red, but when it stagnates, it turns black. Blood nourishes the entire body, and when it does not flow properly, the body becomes malnourished, resulting in a pale complexion and even dehydration. If you see people with such a complexion, you can tell that they have blood circulation problems and are not getting proper nutrition.

The heart controls the vital activities of the human body and is at the top of the list of internal organs. When the heart functions normally, the other five organs work in harmony to promote healthy physiological activities and maintain mental and physical health. However, if the heart develops a pathological condition, the activity of the other organs may become chaotic, leading to mental abnormalities and even endangering life.

b. Liver (肝)

The liver stores blood and regulates blood circulation according to physical activity. If the liver loses its ability to store blood due to disease, one cannot sleep well. The liver also controls the muscles, and its influence is reflected in the nails. Muscle action is movement, and the liver is the source of its nourishment. The liver gives energy to the muscles so that they can move and perform physical activities. The condition of the liver and muscles is always reflected in the nails. People with strong muscles have very strong and thick nails, while people with weak and powerless muscles have thin and fragile nails. When the liver is diseased, the nails become weak, brittle, dry, lose their shine, or may become deformed.

The liver is a constantly active organ, and when the liver Qi (energy) rises too high, a person may become easily angry. Conversely, if the liver Qi is deficient and a person loses his strong and unyielding character, he may become anxious, timid, and develop a smaller gallbladder, making him afraid to take risks.

c. Spleen (脾)

The stomach (胃) is responsible for digestion, while the spleen (脾) absorbs and transports vital fluids to nourish the entire body, making the spleen the foundation of the acquired constitution. Its functions include aiding digestion and assisting in the distribution of vital fluids produced by the stomach. The spleen regulates the body's fat, and its influence is reflected in the lips. When a person's diet is adequate, the body becomes plump with fat. If the spleen becomes diseased, it can cause digestion and absorption problems, leading to weakness in the body and weight loss. A diseased spleen can cause discoloration of the lips, resulting in a yellowish tint and a lack of shine.

The spleen also regulates the extremities. All the limbs receive the nutrients produced by the stomach, and to function properly, they must rely on the spleen's transport function. If the spleen becomes diseased, it cannot transport vital fluids, causing poor circulation in the limbs, resulting in muscle weakness and poor mobility.

The spleen also controls the blood. Blood is made from the essence of grain and water and is produced in the spleen and stomach. Therefore, the spleen has the function of absorbing blood. When the blood-regulating function of the spleen is lost, various bleeding disorders may occur, so the spleen must be nourished to restore blood flow and regulate bleeding disorders.

d. Lungs (肺)

The lungs (肺) are responsible for regulating the skin and hair, as well as facilitating breathing and the exchange of air inside and outside the body. They function by distributing the body's energy and promoting the circulation of Qi through the sweat glands in the skin. The condition of the skin and hair depends on the warmth provided by the lung energy, and if not properly nourished, they can become dry and withered. Lung diseases are reflected in the condition of the skin and hair. When the skin and hair receive pathogenic influences, the disease is transferred to the lungs because the lungs are connected to the skin, and the effects are manifested in the hair.

The lungs (肺) regulate the vital energy of the body, as expressed in the saying "The lungs are the root of Qi." Qi is the source of vital functions in the human body and includes the essence of food and grain as well as the inhalation of natural Qi in the body. Natural Qi is said to have five colors[62]. When Qi enters through the nose, it is transformed into vital energy (氖) and stored in the heart and lungs. As this vital energy rises, it brings a radiant complexion to the face and a strong and clear voice.

---

[62] These five colors are linked to the five elements: Wood is green, Fire is red, Earth is yellow, Metal is white, and Water is black.

The essence of food and grain contains the five tastes[63]. When the five tastes enter through the mouth, they are stored and cooked in the stomach and go through the process of digestion and absorption. The refined essence of the five tastes is then transported to the five major organs, nourishing their vital energy and ensuring their harmonious functioning and proper physiological processes. When the body produces body fluids, the spirit is nourished and revitalized.

Natural Qi is inhaled into the body through the lungs, where it combines with the energy derived from food transformation in the center of the chest and becomes lung energy. It travels via the throat, carries the breath, penetrates the heart veins, and spreads throughout the body. Thus, the lungs are the host for the Qi of the whole body. The heart controls the blood, and the lungs control the Qi. Only when the energy of the lungs is properly expanded and distributed can the fluids of the heart circulate normally. Therefore, the main relationship between the Qi of the lungs and the Qi of the heart is one of mutual benefit.

e. Kidneys (肾)

The kidneys store the essence of life, which is the basic substance for the reproductive functions of both men and women. The essence stored in the kidneys is the essence of the five organs and the six bowels. The most important function of the kidneys is to store this essence.

---

[63] The five tastes correspond to the Five Elements as follows: Wood is sour, Fire is bitter, Earth is sweet, Metal is spicy, and Water is salty.

The kidneys produce and regulate the bones, and the health of the hair is related to the kidneys. The kidneys also produce bone marrow, which fills the bones. Bones grow as a result of the nourishment the marrow. If the bone marrow is not replenished, the bones become weak and brittle.

Hair is the external manifestation of the kidneys, and its nourishment comes from the blood. Blood is formed from the essence of the five organs and the six bowels. Therefore, when the essence of the kidneys is deficient, the bones become weak, and the hair loses its luster. When the essence is abundant and the bone marrow is rich, the mind is healthy and strong, and the hair is shiny.

The kidneys regulate the marrow, which is a kind of fluid in the body. When the marrow enters the stomach, the spleen boils it and sends it to the lungs. When the waste products come out of the lungs, the water goes back to the kidneys. The bone marrow has both clear and cloudy components; the clear component rises as the cloudy component descends. When the clear component rises to the lungs, it becomes Qi. Of the clear components, the clearest rises to nourish the skin and hair, while the less clear descends to the bladder for excretion. The clearest portion of the cloudy part is stored in the kidneys. The fluid in the kidneys is transformed into Qi, which rises to the lungs and is transformed back into water. The water then descends to the kidneys. According to the Somoon section of the <u>Yellow Emperor's Inner Canon</u> (黃帝內經), "Among the earthly Qi (地氣), the upper part belongs to the kidneys (腎), which produce the marrow (髓液)."

The five internal organs, including the heart, liver, spleen, lungs, and kidneys, have an interdependent and restrictive relationship in terms of their physiological functions. For example, the heart and kidneys are interrelated, and the spleen and lungs must work together to maintain the body's normal physiological activities. The lungs regulate Qi, and the heart regulates blood. Together, they maintain the circulation of the body's vital energy. The kidneys are the foundation of the body's innate essence and store the essence of the five organs and six bowels, while the spleen is the origin of the body's acquired essence and transports the nutrients of water and grain to nourish and harmonize the five organs and six bowels.

2. The six bowels (六腑)

The primary function of the six bowels is to receive and digest food and fluids, absorb and distribute the essence, and expel waste and impurities. Unlike the five organs, which store and regulate Qi, the six bowels store nothing and maintain a state of constant flow. According to the Yellow Emperor's Inner Canon (黃帝內經), in the chapter "Discussions on the Differentiation of the five organs" (五臟別論), "They emulate the essence of Heaven, so they neither empty nor hoard. Instead, they absorb the turbid qi of the five organs. They are called the "the palace of transformation and transportation."

The five organs each have five emotional aspects, and the six bowels also have their six emotional states. In "Discussions on Emotions and Nature" (論情性), a chapter of <u>The Great Meaning of the Five Elements</u> (五行大義) by Sogil (蔬吉), it is said:

"When a person likes something, the bladder receives it, and the water flows forward because it likes it. That is why it is called 'good' (好).

When a person is angry, the gallbladder receives it, and the lesser yang channel (少陽) becomes active, causing everything to sprout. This is why it is called 'anger' (怒).

When a person dislikes something, the small intestine receives it, and in summer everything grows and blossoms, including hateful lies. This is why it is called 'bad' (惡).

When a person is joyful, the large intestine receives it, and gold is treasured as something precious that brings joy to everyone. That is why it is called 'joy' (喜).

When a person is happy, the stomach receives it, and the soil produces and nourishes everything, while both the upper and lower parts rejoice. That is why it is called 'happiness' (樂).

When a person is sad, the triple burner receives it, and becomes the abode of yin and yang. Yang rises up and yin settles down. That is why it is called 'sad' (哀)."

The emotion of contentment stimulating the bladder makes sense in terms of its role in regulating water in the body. Similarly, the other six bowels have a deep connection with specific emotions and Jang-Fu organs. Therefore, it is important to consider the six bowels when examining physical symptoms.

a. Gallbladder (膽)

The gallbladder (膽) contains bile (膽汁) and is considered the bowel of the central essence. Its nature is resolute and firm, and when it is strong, it can make decisive judgments. If the gallbladder is affected by pathogenic factors, one may immediately become mentally ill and unable to make decisions. When the bile overflows and rises, a bitter taste appears in the mouth. When the bile refluxes into the stomach, the bile leaks out, causing a bitter taste in the mouth and nausea due to the reverse movement of stomach Qi.

b. Stomach (胃)

The stomach (胃) is responsible for receiving and digesting food and absorbing nutrients, and it is the foundation of the body's vital energy and blood. That is why it is called the sea of vital energy and blood. When the stomach is diseased, it loses its digestive function, and the five organs (五臟) and six bowels (六腑), as well as the four limbs (四肢) and all the bones (百骸), cannot receive nourishment. Therefore, if a person stops eating, he will die, and if there is no stomach pulse (胃氣), he will die.

c. Small Intestine (小腸)

The small intestine (小腸) receives the water and grains (水穀) from the stomach and processes them by distinguishing the clear from the cloudy. The clear substance becomes the essence, and the cloudy substance becomes waste. The clear substance is absorbed and transported to various parts of the body, eventually entering the bladder, while the waste enters the large intestine. When the small intestine is diseased, it cannot differentiate between clear and cloudy substances, resulting in poor absorption and nutrition due to the indiscriminate excretion of substances.

d. Large Intestine (大肠)

The large intestine removes waste and absorbs water. Starting from the top, it receives the leftovers from the small intestine and absorbs water from them before producing feces and sending them down to the rectum. When the colon is diseased, it cannot properly absorb water from waste, leading to diarrhea and dehydration. Symptoms of colon disease include dry stools, abdominal cramps, and diarrhea. When both the stomach and colon are diseased, the symptoms vary depending on whether the stomach is cold or hot and whether the colon is cold or hot. If the stomach is cold, the abdomen will swell, while a cold colon will cause diarrhea. If the stomach is hot and the large intestine and/or colon is cold, the abdomen will swell, diarrhea will occur, and the lower abdomen may hurt.

e. Bladder (膀胱)

The bladder (膀胱) functions to store and eliminate urine and is considered part of the body's fluid and moisture system. When the fluids circulate properly, urine is produced and enters the bladder. If there is a deficiency of fluids, urinary problems may occur, and conversely, if there is an excess of urine, fluids may be lost. Therefore, there is always an interdependent relationship between urine and body fluids.

f. Triple Burner (三焦, Samcho)

The triple burner or Samcho (三焦) is divided into upper burner (上焦; sangcho), middle burner (中焦; jungcho), and lower burner (下焦; hacho.)

Upper Burner (上焦, Sangcho)

The upper burner emerges from the upper opening of the stomach and extends to the chest, piercing the diaphragm. Its functions include accepting food and preventing it from leaving the stomach prematurely. The Sangcho receives the water and grain Qi from the stomach, nourishing the muscles, joints, and skin throughout the body.

Middle Burner (中焦, Jungcho)

The middle burner comes out of the stomach and receives the essence of food and drink, transforming the waste into blood that nourishes the body. Its functions are as follows: It decomposes and cooks food and distills it into body fluids. It absorbs the essence of food and drink to generate and nourish the body's energy.

Lower Burner (下焦, Hacho)

The lower burner function comes from the lower stomach and descends to the bladder. Its function is to distinguish between the good and bad and to excrete waste, as its Qi travels mainly downward.

Thus, the work of the three burners regulates the entire water channel and controls all Qi. The key to maintaining the physiological function of the three burners is the lower burner's Myeongmun (GV4). The three burners receive natural Qi from GV4 and distribute it throughout the body to promote normal activities of organs and tissues.

The six bowels (六腑; Six Fu) include the gallbladder, stomach, large intestine, small intestine, bladder, and triple burner. The process of digestion, absorption of food, and excretion of waste can only be completed when the six bowels function individually as well as in concert.

B. The Non-organ System (奇恒之腑)

Anything in the body that is not an organ can be called a non-organ system. This non-organ system includes the brain, bone marrow, bones, blood vessels, and the uterus. The brain and bone marrow correspond to the modern medical concept of the brain and spinal cord, which make up the central nervous system. Bones, along with muscles, provide the structure that supports the body. The vessels are divided into vessels and collateral vessels, which are further divided into twelve primary vessels and eight extraordinary vessels. The primary vessels correspond to the arterial system, while the collateral vessels correspond to the nervous system. The extraordinary vessels correspond to the venous system. The uterus is a unique feature of females, while it is difficult to find its corresponding feature in men. Although the correspondence between traditional and modern medical concepts may seem somewhat forced, we can simply see it as a difference in perspective between the two approaches and move on.

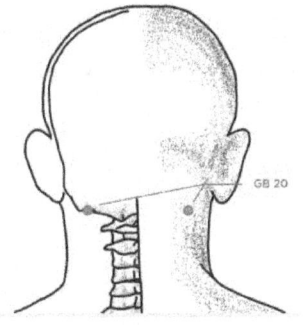

1. Brain (腦)

The brain (腦) is located inside the skull, extending upward to the parietal bones (天靈蓋) and downward to GB20 (風池穴; Gallbladder 20), which is below the spinal cord. The spinal cord is connected to the ventricles of the brain and has a close relationship with the body's bone marrow. All the bone marrow (髓) belongs to the brain, which is why it is called the ocean of bone marrow. The brain controls the movement of the limbs, sharpens the senses, and enables normal mental activity. When the marrow of the brain is abundant, the body feels light and strong, able to perform important tasks with ease. However, when the marrow is depleted, the head becomes cloudy, and one may feel inclined to lie down. The kidneys and the brain are closely related because the kidneys store essence and produce bone marrow. Bone marrow and brain marrow are interdependent. Bone marrow is produced by the kidneys, is stored in the bones, and nourishes the bones.

There is a belief that the brain is related to vitality and reproductive ability. For example, there has been extensive research on drugs that supplement brain marrow, with the idea that abundant brain marrow prevents aging and prolongs life. As a result, there is a technique called restoring essence to the brain (還精補腦), which involves replenishing the brain by returning essence. This technique is one of the methods used in the pursuit of immortality and longevity in the methods of cultivating life. It involves bringing the essence into the brain through the spinal canal (intrathecal), and it is important to vividly visualize the specific image in one's mind. This is because such visualization helps to track and draw the essence upward.

2. Marrow (髓)

The marrow is generated by the kidneys (腎) and is stored in the bones, providing nourishment to the bones. The bone marrow (骨髓)

within the bones is closely related to brain marrow through the bone cavities (骨空).

3. Bones (骨)

Bones play a role in supporting and maintaining the structure of the body. They receive nutrients from the bone marrow to maintain their health. While bones can store bone marrow, they cannot produce it on their own and must rely on the kidneys, which are the site of bone marrow production. Without adequate production of bone marrow by the kidneys, bones cannot become strong and solid.

4. Vessels (脈)

The vessels are closely related to the heart. The vessels belong to the heart; the vessels are also part of the blood all of which are considered the conduit for Qi. The vessels and heart have a mutually beneficial relationship and are interdependent. The vessels are capable of transporting both blood and Qi and are able to regulate and maintain the flow of both in a consistent and harmonious manner. The vessels are distributed throughout the body and serve to transport blood and nutrients, while also assisting in the purification of food.

C. Harmonizing the Internal Organs (臟腑)

The organs (臟) store essence of life (Jeong) (精) and Qi, while the bowels control the transformation and transportation of food essence. Therefore, the five organs belong to the Yin category, and the six bowels belong to the Yang category. The Yang organs govern the outside, and the Yin organs govern the inside. The combination of an organ and an bowel, a yin and a yang, and an inside and an outside form a functional unit called the organ-bowel combination.

D. Internal Organs (臟腑) and the Nine Outlets (九竅)

The eyes (目), mouth (口), ears (耳), nose (鼻), and tongue (舌) are collectively called the five sense organs (五官) or the seven orifices (七竅). The seven orifices refers to the seven openings or cavities on the human head, which include the eyes, ears, nostrils, and mouth. Together with the front (前陰; urethra) and back (後陰; anus) openings, they are called the nine orifices (九竅). Although the internal organs are located inside the body, they have a close relationship and alignment with the sense organs and orifices (五官九竅).

1. The Ears (耳)

The Ears (耳) and the Kidneys

The kidneys (腎) store the essence (精) and produce the marrow (髓), which is connected to the brain. When the brain is relaxed and abundant, the ears (耳) become sharp and clear, but when the brain is deficient, the ears may feel blocked or dull. Finally, the harmonious flow of kidney Qi (腎氣) gives the ears the capacity to hear the five sounds (五音)[64] effectively.

The Ears (耳) and the Heart (心)

The heart (心) controls the circulation of blood. For the ears (耳) to function properly in terms of hearing, there must be a sufficient supply of Qi and blood. If there is a deficiency of Qi and blood in the vessels, the ears will quickly become sensitive, resulting in abnormal hearing.

The Ears (耳) and the Liver-Gallbladder (肝膽)

The liver (肝) and the gallbladder (膽) regulate the upward and outward movement of Qi. If there is a deficiency in the upward and outward movement of Qi, the upper part of the body will be deficient, resulting in a stuffy feeling in the ears. If there is an excess of Qi in the upward movement, the upper part of the body will be excessively active, resulting in tinnitus (ringing in the ears).

---

[64]Five Sounds (五音): In Daoism, the five sounds or five tones are associated with the five elements (wood, fire, earth, metal, and water) and the corresponding musical notes in the Chinese pentatonic scale: Gong, Shang, Jue, Zhi, and Yu. These sounds are integral to various aspects of Taoist philosophy and practice.

2. The Eyes (目)

The Eyes (目) and the Liver (肝)

The eyes (目) are considered the orifices (竅) of the liver (肝). The liver stores blood (血) and is responsible for the upward and outward movement of Qi (升發). If there is not enough blood in the liver, it can lead to decreased visual acuity. If the upward movement of liver Qi is excessive, it can cause redness and bloodshot eyes. When the liver is in a harmonious state, it enables the ability to see the five colors (五色).

The Eyes (目) and the Heart (心腸)

The heart is the owner of the blood vessels, so the eyes can only see when they are supplied with Qi and blood from the heart.

The Eyes (目) and the Internal Organs (臟腑)

The essential Qi of the five Jang[65] and six Fu[66] is sent through the blood vessels to the two eyes and becomes the essence of the eyes. The eyes are the dwelling place of the essence, where all stability is maintained. The eyes are divided into left and right, where the left is yang and the right is yin. The left is Fu, and the right is Jang. The eye consists of the eyeball, pupil, iris, sclera, conjunctiva, eyelid, and lacrimal gland.

---

[65] Five Jang include: the liver, heart, spleen, lung, and kidneys.
[66] Six Fu include: the gallbladder, small intestine, stomach, large intestine, bladder, and triple burner.

The correspondence between the eyes and the Jang-Fu organs is shown in the following table:

왼쪽 눈 Left eye	부(腑) Fu (six bowels)	오른쪽 눈 Right eye	장(臟) Jang (five organs)
눈동자(瞳) Pupil	방광 Urinary bladder	눈동자(瞳) Pupil	신장 Kidneys
안흑(眼黑) Iris	담 Gallbladder	안흑(眼黑) Iris	간장 Liver
안피(眼皮) Conjunctiva	위 Stomach	안피(眼皮) Conjunctiva	비장 Spleen
안각(眼殼) Lacrimal gland	소장 Small intestine	안각(眼殼) Lacrimal gland	심장 Heart
안백(眼白) Sclera	대장 Large intestine	안백(眼白) Sclera	폐 Lungs

3. The Nose (鼻)

The Nose (鼻) and the Lungs (肺)

The nose (鼻) is the gateway for breathing. The lungs (肺) are responsible for breathing. Therefore, the nose is the bright aperture of the lungs. The nose can detect odors, but normal olfactory function requires harmonious lung Qi and smooth breathing. If the lung Qi is deficient, the nose may become congested and not function properly.

4. The Mouth (口)

The spleen (脾) is responsible for digestion, and when the spleen is functioning well, it sends out hunger signals that make a person feel the desire to eat. The energy of the spleen is connected to the mouth, and when the spleen is in harmony, the mouth can distinguish the flavors of different grains. The mouth is the bright aperture of the spleen. The Foot Yangming (足陽明) is the channel of the Stomach and Intestines, connects to the mouth, surrounds the lips, and wraps around the inside the mouth.

5. The Tongue (舌)

The tongue (舌) controls taste, and taste is where the Qi of the heart (心氣) flows. Qi flows through the tongue, so when the heart is working harmoniously, the tongue can discern taste well. However, if the Qi of the heart is disharmonious, one may not be able to taste food properly even when eating it. So, the tongue is the master of the heart's sensory perception. The heart and the small intestine are related in a way called the "outer-inner" relationship. Therefore, when the small intestine is too hot, the tongue becomes red, and symptoms such as sores on the tongue may occur. In addition, the three major vessels, the liver (肝), spleen (脾), and kidneys (腎), all communicate with the tongue. Therefore, diseases of the liver, spleen, and kidneys are often associated with the tongue.

6. The Anterior Perineum (前陰)

The Anterior Perineum (前陰) and the Kidneys (腎)

When the renal artery (腎脈) becomes slippery and enlarged, it is a symptom of renal fever (腎熱症), and if there is a bladder stone, urine does not come out cool like it should, but instead causes severe pain.

The Anterior Perineum (前陰) and the Liver (肝)

The vessels of the liver circulate Yin energy throughout the body, such as in the flow of the Jueyin liver meridian of the foot (足厥陰). The anterior perineum is the gathering point of the perineal muscle, and there is a significant relationship between the anterior perineum and the liver.

Interaction between the Anterior Perineum (前陰) and other Organs and Bowels (腸腑)

When the spleen vessel is weak and slippery, it is a symptom of heat in the spleen and intestines. When the heat descends to the anterior perineum, it causes lower abdominal pain and urinary retention. The kidney, bladder, spleen, stomach, liver, and conception & governor vessels all have a relationship with the anterior perineum.

7. The Posterior Perineum (後陰)

The anus is primarily associated with the kidneys and lungs. If the function of the kidney meridian is weak and not smooth, it can lead to disorders related to the circulation of Qi and blood. This can result in the absence of menstrual periods as well as conditions such as anal fistulas and bedsores. The lungs and large intestine have a surface-to-internal relationship. The anus is at the end of the large intestine. Hence, individuals with lung heat often experience difficulty in bowel movements, which can lead to the formation of hemorrhoids.

The nine orifices are always related to the five organs, the six bowels, and the twelve vessels. The purpose of classifying them into the five organs is to associate each orifice with its corresponding organ, making it easier to distinguish between the primary and secondary symptoms and to identify the key point.

Part II. Golden Rishi Qigong Training

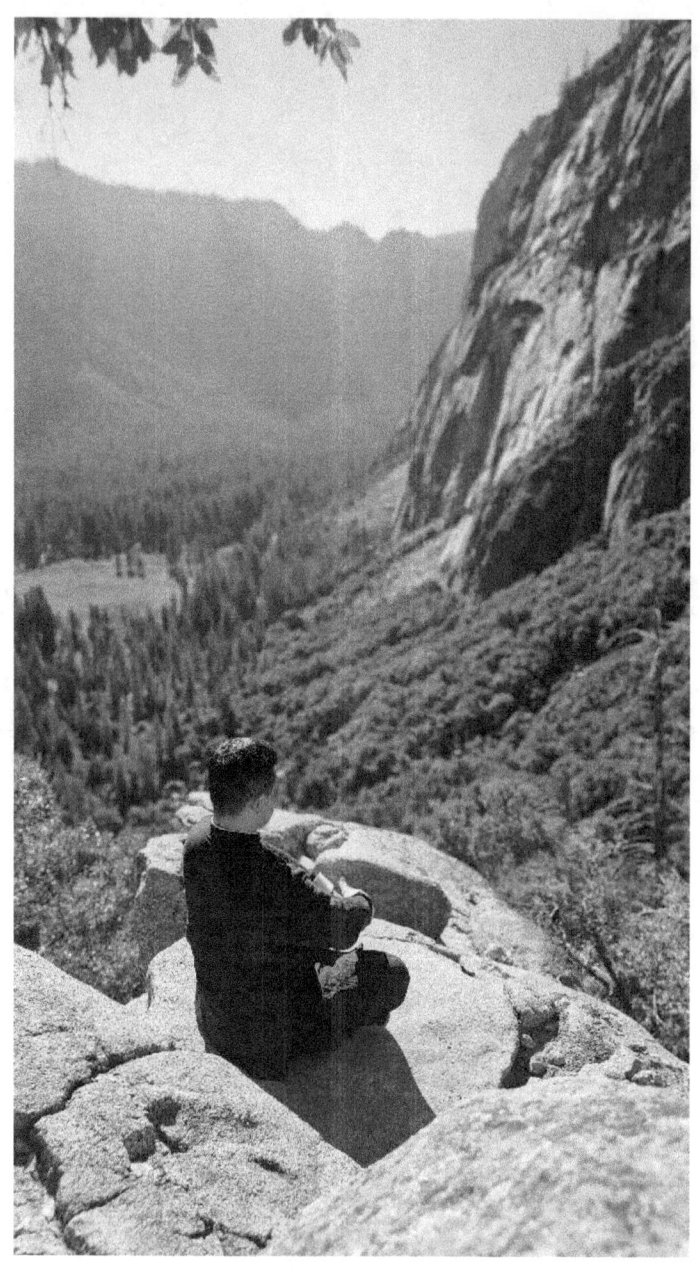

Chapter VI. Course of Practice

The first section of this book contains essential knowledge necessary for training. This chapter builds on that foundational knowledge and describes basic exercises of the Golden Rishi Qigong.

The <u>Inner Canon of the Yellow Emperor</u> [67](黃帝內經) contains a chapter titled, "SuWen: Discussion of Heavenly Truth in Ancient Times" (素問, 上古天地論) in which the Emperor asks, "Is the reason why people can't have children as they age due to the exhaustion of their reproductive ability (材力), or is it due to their predetermined lifespan?"

Qi Bo[68] replied, "At the age of seven, a girl's kidney energy matures, leading to the growth of teeth and hair. At the age of 14, TianGui (天癸)[69] becomes active, the Conception Vessel opens, and TaiChongMai (太冲脉)[70] matures, marking the beginning of menstruation. At the age of 21, the kidney energy is fully developed, and the wisdom teeth grow. At 28, the muscles and bones are fully developed, the hair grows to its maximum length, and the body is in its prime. At 35, however, YangMingMai[71](阳明脉) begins to decline, the face begins to wrinkle,

---

[67] The "Huangdi Neijing" (Yellow Emperor's Inner Canon) is an ancient Chinese medical text that has been foundational in traditional Chinese medicine (TCM) for over two millennia.

[68] Qi Bo, a mythological Chinese doctor, served as a minister to the Yellow Emperor.

[69] TianGui; 天癸: growth and development of the human body

[70] TaiChongMai (太冲脉): the vital channel flowing from the uterus, which is also known as the "Blood Chamber" and "Sea of Blood.".

[71] YangMingMai (阳明脉): One of twelve meridian/pathway known to have abundant Qi and blood flowing. YangMing is associated with the stomach and large intestine. Mai referring to "meridian."

and hair begins to fall out. At 42, the three yang channels in the body decline from top to bottom, the face becomes completely wrinkled, and the hair begins to turn gray. At 49, the Conception Vessel (任脉), known as the "Sea of Yin Channels," is exhausted, the TaiChongMai (太冲脉) shrinks, the TianQui (天癸) dries up, and the Earth Path (地道; connection to earthly things) becomes impassable, leading to physical decline and the inability to bear children."

"At the age of eight years, a boy's kidney Qi begins to fill, causing his hair to grow and his teeth to change. At the age of 16, his kidney Qi is fully developed, reaching the TianGui (天癸), and his vital essence overflows. The harmony of yin and yang enables him to father a child. At 24, his kidney Qi is balanced, his muscles and bones are strong, and his wisdom teeth grow, marking his peak physical growth. At 32, his muscles and bones are at their most robust, and his flesh is firm. At 40, his kidney Qi begins to decline, his hair starts to fall out, and his teeth weaken. At 48, his yang Qi declines from its peak, his face becomes pale, and his hair and beard turn white. At 56, his liver Qi declines, his muscles become less mobile, and at 64, his TianGui (天癸) dries up, his vital essence decreases, and his kidneys weaken. His physique reaches its limit, and his teeth and hair fall out. The kidneys, which govern water, store the vital essence received from the five organs and the six bowels. When the five viscera are full, they can ejaculate, but now that all the five viscera have declined, the muscles and bones become loose. The TianGui is exhausted, his hair and beard turn white, his body becomes heavy, and his gait is not straight, so he cannot have children."

The emperor asked, "Why do some people still have children in their old age?"

Qi Bo replied, "It is because their vital essence remains even after they have passed the Heavenly Number (天壽; a term referring to a predetermined life span or destiny), but even those who have children cannot go beyond the age of 64 for men and 49 for women, after which the vital essence of heaven and earth completely dries up."

The Emperor asked, "Can a person who follows the Dao[72] (道; The Way) have children even after he is over 100 years old?"

Qi Bo replied, "A person who follows the Dao remains physically intact even in old age, and although his body ages he can still have children."

The above discussion explains the physiological processes of human growth, aging, and the onset and disappearance of reproductive ability. Daoists classify human beings into five categories: infant body, leaky body, broken body, declining body, and weak body. Men under the age of 16 and women under the age of 14, referred to as child bodies, can practice the ascension method directly without the need for Qi accumulation training. When males reach 16 and females reach 14, they reach their TianGui (天癸) and begin to produce sperm and eggs, respectively, and are considered leaky bodies. To practice as a leaky body, one must first do the return and accumulation of Qi before practicing the cultivation method of ascension.

---

[72] The Dao is the core principle underlying the universe--ineffable, formless, and transcendent. Harmony with the Dao is considered essential for a balanced and fulfilling life.

When men and women copulate and have children, they become broken bodies. To cultivate with a broken body, you have to solidify your essence and blood, repair the leaky body, go back to the origin, accumulate Qi, and return it to the child's body before you start the cultivation method.

At the age of 56 for men and 42 for women, people reach the stage of a declining body, and at the age of 64 for men and 49 for women, you reach the stage of a weak body. To practice as a weak body or a declining body, one must first use all his strength to steal the purification of heaven and earth to repair the weak body, accumulate yang to increase vitality, solidify essence and blood, repair the leaky body, and return and accumulate Qi to return to the infant body, and then he can practice the cultivation way.

In other words, as human beings go through the process of growth and decay, our bodies inevitably weaken. The practice of Golden Rishi Qigong can reverse this process, restore health, and allow us to enjoy our heavenly lifespan (天数; to live to our predestined age and not die before then from illness). The process of refining the body and absorbing Qi is considered a very important step in the overall restoration of health.

The practice of Golden Rishi Qigong is divided into five stages. When one practices Stage 1: Refining the Body and Cultivating Qi and Stage 2: Refining the Essence and Transforming Qi, one completes the

Mao-You Jucheon[73] (卯酉周天) and the Sojucheon[74] (小周天; Microcosmic Orbit). This leads to the realization of general health practice and the pursuit of the Dao (道; the Way) in daily life. The study beyond "Refining Qi and Transforming Spirit" depends on the practitioner's aptitude, enthusiasm, level of practice, family karma, and other personal circumstances and environmental factors that determine whether he can progress further.

Stage 1. Refining the Body and Cultivating Qi (煉身攝氣)

- Dispels disease, preserves life, and improves physical health.
- Facilitates the flow of vessels and regulates the balance of Yin and Yang.
- Replenishes the leakage, establishes the foundation, and returns to the origin.

Through Wood Meditation (平衡功; the practice of balancing, exchanging Qi with trees), Sleep Meditation (睡功; sleeping skill), Walking Meditation (自然換氣法; the practice of walking, exchanging Qi with nature), and the Human Immortal Method (人仙法), one cultivates all postures of walking, standing, moving, sitting, and lying down. By absorbing what is clear and diligently expelling what is cloudy, one cultivates the foundation of the body and preserves the essence of life.

---

[73] Mao-You Jucheon practice aligns with the time periods of Mao (dawn) and You (dusk).

[74] Sojucheon "小周天" (Xiǎo Zhōutiān(CN), translates to "Microcosmic Orbit" in English. It refers to a specific energetic path in Taoist and Chinese energy practices that directs the circulation of vital energy (qi) in the body.

Stage 2. Refining Essence and Transforming Qi (煉精化氣)

- All pathogenic energies are unable to cause harm, leading to a state of tranquility with minimal disease.
- Being peaceful and content while experiencing joy leads to a disease-free state and an extension of one's life span.
- Extending one's life span and enjoying longevity, fully experiencing the blessings of a long life.

By completing the Mao You Orbit (卯酉周天; the circulation of vital energy between heaven and earth) and the Sojucheon (Microcosmic Orbit), one enters the stage of the spiritual realm. Through dedicated seated meditation practice, one harmonizes the internal and external vital energy (精; essence and 气; energy) within the human body, forming an internal cosmic structure composed of Qi. Internally, one becomes aware of various energetic pathways and dynamic formations, while externally, one senses and interacts with the Qi and its manifestations outside the body, gaining a complete understanding of the body.

Stage 3. Refining Qi and Transforming Spirit (鍊氣化神)

- Prolongs life, increases longevity, and returns to youthfulness from old age.
- Through the practice of refining the physical form, one attains longevity and vitality that can last a thousand years.
- By cultivating extreme Yang energy, the body becomes light, and the mind becomes agile.

By completing the Daejucheon (大周天; Macrocosmic Orbit), one reaches the stage of earthly immortality (地仙公), focusing on the practice of sitting meditation. By harmonizing Qi and mind internally and externally within the cosmic structure of the human body, one transforms and returns to the innate divine form. Internally, one becomes aware of the movement patterns of the pre- and posthumous spirits. Externally, one senses the changes in the earth's atmosphere and gains a deep awareness of the connection between heaven and earth. This leads to a transformation of the yin and yang aspects of life and the attainment of longevity.

Stage 4. Cultivating the Spirit and Return to Emptiness (鍊神還虛)

- Refining the form to cultivate Qi, which endures throughout eternity.
- Refining the spirit to encompass emptiness and embrace receptiveness so life's experiences naturally flow in and out of one harmoniously.
- Transcending the ordinary and entering the realm of the sacred, returning to the three paths.[75](三道)

By corresponding to the realm of Heavenly Immortality (天仙功), with the practice of sitting meditation at its core, one refines the mind within the cosmic structure of the human body and transforms it into

---

[75] The Three Path refers to the three stages of practice widely recognized in Theravada and Mahayana Buddhism: insight, practice, and non-possession.

emptiness. The formless becomes form, and the formless essence becomes tangible. Internally, one attains self-realization of the origin of life and death, while externally, one perceives the atmospheric conditions of the solar system, gaining a profound understanding of the universe and harmonizing all things. This stage leads back to the state of primordial chaos and attains for the practitioner eternal life.

Stage 5. Cultivating Emptiness and Harmonizing with the Dao (鍊虛合道)

- Reaching emptiness and boundlessness, where both exist without limitation.
- Activating and transforming Qi, profound and mysterious in its subtlety.
- The twenty-eight constellations are all in the realm of repentance that most spiritual and philosophical traditions have where the person makes amends for previous actions.
- Cultivating emptiness is in line with the Dao, establishing the foundation and returning to the source. This is the stage of integration.

In particular, the process of Stage #1: Refining the Body and Cultivating Qi (煉身攝氣), is the process of shaping the body. Through Golden Rishi Qigong basic training one learns various cultivation methods, such as sleep meditation (睡功), wood meditation (平衡功, the practice of balance, exchanging Qi with trees), walking meditation (自然換氣法; the walking practice, exchanging Qi with nature), Sun Meditation (盜日精歸己法, method of withdrawing the essence of the sun and returning it to oneself), Moon Meditation (盜月華歸己法, method of withdrawing the brilliance of the moon and returning it to oneself). After developing a strong foundation and finding places with abundant vital energy, one engages in outdoor training in the mountains and absorbs natural Qi. Only after the physical body has been built through this process does one enter the cultivation of Stage 2: Refining the Essence and Transforming Qi (煉精化氣).

This section contains many aspects recorded in the book Secret Transmission of Master Zhongli's Complete "Methods of the Sacred Jewel (靈寶畢法)[76]". However, for those who are new to the practice, it is advisable to start with the basics under the guidance of a proper master. This will enable one to cultivate properly without having to make unnecessary trials and errors.

Chapter VII. Seated Meditation

A. Sitting Posture

When a person is in the mother's womb, the lowest point is that of the two sciatic nerves, and the highest point is the head. Practitioners should consider reversing their acquired (postnatal) state to their

---

[76] The Methods of the Sacred Jewel is a Taoist text dating back to the late Tang or Five Dynasties period. It is included in the Daoist Canon under the section of the Supreme Purity and is also known as Zhongli's Transmission to Lü Dongbin of the Complete Methods of the Sacred Jewel. Attributed to Zhongli Quan and Lü Dongbin, legendary figures in Taoism and among the Eight Immortals, it delves into the practice of internal alchemy aimed at achieving immortality through refining internal energy.

innate (prenatal) state. Initially, one imitates the shape of the innate state by half-sitting, and then transforms into the form of the innate state. Half-sitting is divided into three types: natural sitting posture, half-lotus sitting posture, and lotus sitting posture. Since lotus sitting posture can only be achieved after considerable practice, Golden Rishi sitting posture is a compromise between half lotus sitting posture and lotus sitting posture and is recommended.

1. Natural Sitting Posture

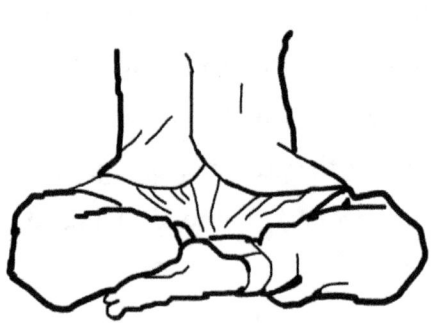

This seated method is also called the completed sitting, similar to the Siddhasana [77] in Yoga. The right heel is placed tightly against the perineum, and the left heel is placed against the right ischium, the bottom of the pelvis. The left foot is not placed on the right foot or right leg. The important thing here is to keep the spine straight. Force is applied to the 4th and 5th lumbar vertebra, pushing as much as possible towards the front of the body. This allows the sacrum (the bone at the base of the spine) to stand upright. The most important thing in all seated methods is to keep the sacrum vertical. This method blocks the KD1 [78] （涌泉 acupoint) on both legs. This

---

[77] Siddhasana is a seated yoga pose that is often referred to as the "accomplished" or "perfect" pose.
[78] Yongcheon refers to a specific acupuncture point, Kidney 1 (K1), located on the sole of the foot.

posture has four points of support: two sciatic nerves and two legs, but the posture is a bit unstable.

2. Half Lotus Sitting Posture

This seating method is commonly referred to as the half-lotus sitting posture. It doesn't matter whether you lift your left foot or your right foot. The important thing is to choose the side that is comfortable for you. One leg is placed on the root of the thigh of the other leg. The upper leg presses down on the lower leg, tensioning the KD1 (涌泉 acupoint) and the thigh muscle. This posture has three points of support: two sciatic nerves and one leg. This posture is relatively stable.

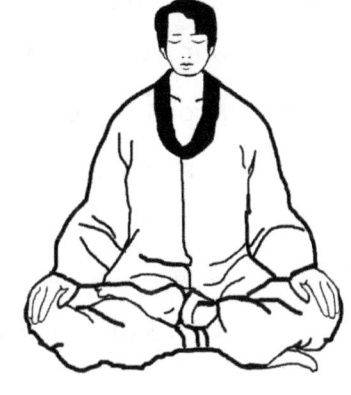

Some books divide the left and right sides into yin and yang, but in reality, this has little effect on healthy people. Usually, people find it comfortable to lift their left foot. If your legs become numb from sitting for a long time, it is fine to switch sides.

3. Golden Rishi Sitting Posture

In this seated method, the right heel is also placed against the perineum. For men, since the scrotum is in front of the perineum, it is

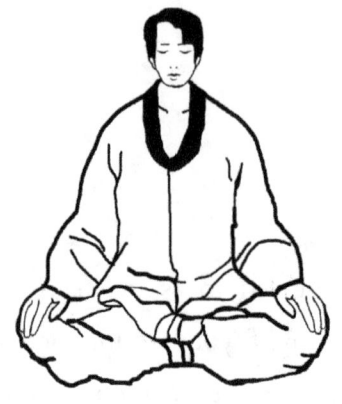

necessary to lift the scrotum with your hand first, place the heel against the perineum, and then release your hand to place the scrotum inside the right heel. Then, the left foot is placed on the right leg, but the foot is inserted between the calf and the thigh, shaped like a knife blade. Be careful not to place it on your thigh. Both knees should touch the ground. If you bring your left foot too close to your right knee, your left knee will lift off the ground. This seated method also requires you to apply force to the GV4[79] (命门; lower back) and keep the sacrum upright.

4. Lotus Sitting Posture

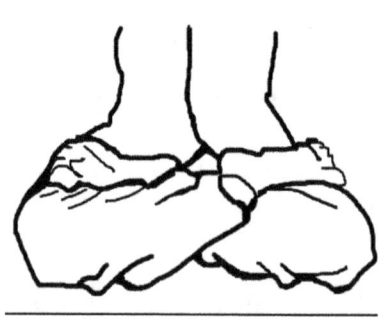

This sitting posture, also known as the full lotus posture or the lotus sitting posture, is the most challenging posture. It takes practice, effort, and patience to achieve this posture correctly. In

---

[79] Myeongmun (命门, GV4) is located on the lower back, specifically in the region between the second and third lumbar vertebrae. It is found on the spine, opposite the navel.

yoga, this posture is also considered the ultimate asana. All other asanas are considered to be preparatory stages for achieving this posture. Initially, the name of this posture changes depending on whether you lift your right foot first or last.

Most people find it easier to lift their right foot first. This posture is called anti-evil sitting (降魔坐). Conversely, the action of putting the left foot first is called auspicious sitting (吉祥坐). After attaining enlightenment, the Buddha is said to have moved from anti-evil sitting to auspicious sitting. However, it is unclear whether this change has any meaning beyond its symbolic implications. In the Kagyu school[80] of Vajrayana (also known as Esoteric Buddhism), practitioners adopt the auspicious posture.

Vajrayana[81] (also known as Esoteric Buddhism) aims to achieve Buddhahood in this very body and life, hence the adoption of such a posture. In any case, the practitioner should begin with the posture that is easiest for him or her. In most cases, the anti-evil (降魔坐) posture is easier, but if someone finds the auspicious (吉祥坐) posture more comfortable, they might be a unique case and may have practiced Vajrayana Buddhism in a previous life.

Let's take the example of a relatively common posture, the anti-evil sitting posture (降魔坐). When lifting your right foot, it is best to keep your left leg as straight as possible. The reason for this is to establish

---

[80] The Kagyu school is a notable Tibetan Buddhist tradition known for its emphasis on direct transmission of teachings and practical meditation guidance from teacher to student.

[81] Vajrayana, also called Tantric Buddhism, is a diverse tradition within Buddhism focused on rituals, meditation practices, and esoteric techniques for attaining enlightenment.

the habit of placing your right foot as low as possible so that the toes of your right foot extend beyond the outer line of your left thigh when you first form the full lotus posture (跏趺坐). Beginners can probably touch the floor with their right knee in this position.

After your right foot is in place, it is important to quickly lift your left foot and place it so that the toes of your left foot extend even further beyond the outer line of your right thigh. The reason for crossing your legs so deeply is to protect your right ankle.

If you're going to be sitting for a long time (over an hour), it is important to cross your legs deeply; otherwise, you run the risk not only of ankle pain but also of stretching the ligaments in your ankle.

The most important aspect of this sitting meditation (坐法) is to keep your sacrum (薦骨) upright. Typically, the joints in the GV4 area (命門, also known as the "Gate of Life") recede due to pain, but if this happens, it is better not to do this posture. If you can keep your spine straight while doing this posture correctly, various new phenomena will occur in your body. The blocked Qi cavities (氣穴) in the conception vessel and the governing vessel (任督脈) are stimulated, causing vibrations or slight pain. However, these are all mere healing crises (瞑眩反應) and are not overly worrisome. Not only do these Qi cavity pathways (氣穴) open up, but the Sojucheon (microcosmic orbit) and the elixir circuit (丹道) happen much more easily.

Ultimately, these sitting methods are all designed to align the spine and properly stimulate kundalini, or the Refining Essence and Transforming Qi (煉精化氣). To facilitate these methods, it is essential to practice all forms of Dao Yin techniques[82]. Although there are some people who are born with special bodies that have supple joints, aligned vertebrae like a child, and sacral bones that are divided into segments, this book is not intended for them. Such individuals naturally possess all the necessary practices in their subconscious and don't need external teachings. However, most practitioners who aren't so naturally gifted have to make great efforts and endure hardships to discipline their physical bodies. This physical discipline leads to the unity of mind and body (心身合一). It is like taming a wild horse- only when it is trained can it realize its potential. In the same way, people who are born with healthy bodies often don't take care of them and may have shorter lives. In contrast, many great masters of internal martial arts and other disciplines overcame weak and sickly bodies in their youth. Their sweat and tears elevated them to mastery. Qigong (氣功) is not just a hobby for fame; it becomes a path to the illumination of one's true essence and a means of attaining longevity and eternal youth (不老長生) when it is transformed into a practice under the discipline of Seon Do (仙道). Therefore, those who desire fruitful results should practice diligently and not neglect their training.

B. Breathing Methods

People generally think that the Dantian (丹田; elixir field) is located about three fingers' distance below the navel and two-thirds of the way

---

[82] Dao Yin techniques are traditional Qigong exercises that involve body movements and stretching to promote the flow of energy (Qi).

inside the body. Although it is not incorrect to think of this as the location of the Dantian, the term "Dantian" actually refers to a field where the elixir (丹) is present, so in reality, the entire lower abdomen corresponds to the Dantian.

On the other hand, the Qi cavity (氣穴) refers to the "cave" or "pouch" of Qi, and its location varies slightly between men and women. For women, it corresponds to the location of the uterus, and for men, it corresponds to the location of the testicles. The supporting organs are the ovaries in women and the prostate in men and are associated with the hormone glands that secrete the essence of life (Jeong). The hormone glands are closely related to nerve cells and resonate with nerve activity throughout the body. Therefore, whenever an action is taken, there is immediate feedback that maintains harmony.

We operate our bodies by circulating and transforming Qi in this Qi cavity (氣穴). In order to do this, breathing methods are very important.

There are many different breathing methods, but let's choose one that is relatively effective and has no side effects at the stage of Refining the Essence and Transforming Qi (煉精化氣). In typical cases, practitioners try certain actions while holding their breath, hoping for quick results. However, there are many instances where the side effects are so severe that further cultivation becomes impossible. In order to avoid such side effects, it is necessary to engage in rigorous physical training, similar to those dedicated practitioners who retreat to secluded mountains and valleys. In today's practical reality, where such conditions are almost impossible, it is advisable to practice breathing techniques in addition to doing physical exercises. Therefore, I would like to introduce breathing techniques that minimize side effects while being relatively effective.

● Stage 1

When inhaling, contract the sphincter muscle. Any posture is acceptable, whether standing, sitting, walking, or lying down. The issue at this stage is to start training to contract the sphincter muscle, so the more it is done the better.

● Stage 2

Inhale and contract the anal sphincter only at the pause after one stop inhaling, but before the exhalation. Next, exhale with the sphincter still contracted. After exhaling, release the sphincter, stop breathing for a moment and contract the sphincter again.

This is a bit difficult for beginners. It is best to do it sitting down, and remember, as with all meditation, it is important to keep the spine upright when sitting.

● Stage 3

Here we do the opposite of Stage 1 and contract the sphincter muscle while exhaling and relax the sphincter muscle while inhaling. It is not easy to contract the sphincter muscle when exhaling, as this is the moment when the body loses strength. But with practice, one can achieve it. It is also important to do this while sitting first. If one does not straighten the waist, the muscles in the perineal area cannot be activated. The order of the breathing method and contracting the sphincter muscle is completely opposite to Stage 1, so it may be difficult to learn at first, but afterwards one will contract the perineal area whenever one continues to exhale. This is necessary for the correct Dantian breathing (丹田呼吸) to occur.

● **Stage 4**

During exhalation, contract the anal sphincter. After completely exhaling, hold the breath and focus on the perineum, pulling it in toward the tailbone of the spine, imagining that the perineum is bumping into the tip of the tailbone. When one becomes short of breath, breathe in, releasing the perineum and sphincter. Remember to keep the back straight.

● **Stage 5**

Repeat the process of pulling and hitting the tailbone with the perineum several times while in the fully exhaled state of Stage 4. This usually takes about 10 to 20 times. Then, when one becomes out of breath, relax the sphincter while inhaling. For a fast and powerful hit, it is fine if the back bends slightly. Stage 5 is particularly used for gathering energy or as an auxiliary means to strengthen the perineum muscles, and in regular practice, the breathing of stage 4 is the main focus.

● **Stage 6**

In the breathing of Stage 5, regardless of inhaling or exhaling, continuously and rapidly repeat the process of tensing and relaxing the sphincter, aiming to sensitize the muscles of the perineum. Stage 6 is a practice method that can be performed during daily life and can be carried out in any state of movement or rest, whether speaking or silent.

● **Stage 7**

The breath in this stage is the completion breath. Here, one can actually feel the lower Dantian Qi cavity (氣穴) as if it were a single round rubber ball, expanding like a pouch when upon inhalation and collapsing upon exhalation. The breathing method is divided into three steps, the same as in stage 4. The difference is that after fully exhaling, the Qi (氣) in the lower Dantian Qi cavity (氣穴) is raised through the governor vessel. When it reaches the top end of the governor vessel at the crown of the head, known as the GV20 (百會), one inhales. While inhaling, the Qi descends through the conception vessel (任脉) and sends the Qi back down into the Lower Dantian Qi cavity (氣穴).

As one exhales again, you contract your sphincter muscle, and the Qi in the deflating Qi cavities (氣穴) pouch passes through the tailbone of the GV1 (長強穴; tailbone) to the base of the spine (尾閭關). The base of the spine is one of the three major Qi cavities (氣穴) in the Governor vessel. After fully exhaling, you enter a state of breath retention, drawing the Qi located in the base of the spine up to GV20 (百會) through the governor vessel. As it rises, you should feel a sense of warmth, and this heat cools in the palace of Nirvana (泥丸宮; the pineal gland, which is located in the brain), turning into cool water. It feels as if a kind of condensation is occurring. As you inhale again, you expand the pouch of the lower Dantian's Qi cavity, open your sphincter muscle, and send the gathered Qi at the top of the head down again through the Conception vessel. This Qi transforms as if it were a cool stream of water, entering the pouch of the lower Dantian. At this point, you feel the Dantian cooling down.

In this way, a cycle of the Conception and Governor vessels is formed through the three-step process of exhaling (呼), pausing (止), and inhaling (吸). This seventh stage of breathing is indeed the completed breathing method, so one should primarily adhere to this breathing. However, occasionally, it is necessary to practice pausing while holding your breath. At that time, a different flavor is added.

For beginners, there's a risk that holding the breath while inhaling may cause a rise in Qi (上氣) in the Conception vessel, but for those who have reached a certain level of mastery in breathing exercises and are practicing the seven-stage breathing, holding the breath in the state of inhalation can bring a sense of enjoyment in practice. Furthermore, a slight elevation of Qi can be quite interesting for those who have the ability to control it.

The nature of this enjoyment is something one must experience personally. Conversely, these breathing methods fall under the category of 'Musik Breathing,' which means consciously controlled and intentional breathing. 'Munsik Breathing,' on the other hand, is natural and unconscious breathing that is allowed to flow without artificial interference. Munsik Breathing is primarily used as a breathing technique in advanced stages to promote stillness and tranquility. There are occasions when embracing Munsik Breathing becomes essential.

At the stage of Refining the Essence and Transforming Qi (煉精化氣), intentional breathing is mainly used. However, once the "true seed of Dan" is cultivated, natural breathing is mainly practiced. Occasionally, intentional breathing is done when necessary. In Refining Qi and Transforming Spirit (鍊氣化神), natural breathing is the main focus of practice.

Each person's aptitude for the seven stages of the breathing process will vary, but you should try to practice all of them for as little as a week or two or as long as a month or two. This will allow you to fully enjoy the flavors of each stage. This will be very helpful when you teach others in the future, as you will be able to listen to their experiences and judge their physical condition.

Regardless, as we master each of these stages of breathing, we begin to rediscover our senses for our own bodies. Not only do we discover various sensations that we've lost, but we also gain control over our autonomic nervous system. This process is the very embodiment of mind-body unity. If we're deaf to the sounds our body makes, we pass through life unaware of what's happening inside of us, and we'll never achieve unity of mind and body. In the unity of mind and body, the mind inevitably takes the lead, but how can unity be achieved if we ignore or are insensitive to the voices of our body?

Breathing has two main purposes. The first is to produce "Sari" (舍利) in the Dantian. "Sari" is essentially a seed, also called "Jinjongja" (眞種子; true seed) in this context. The most important aspect is the concept of consciousness. Consciousness is a form of divine or spiritual energy, so it is characterized by the properties of fire, referred to as "Shinhwa" (神火) or "divine fire. When this "Shinhwa" combines with the "water" or essence of the kidneys, it forms "sari," which prevents any wasteful dissipation of energy.

The second purpose of breathing is to awaken the Kundalini. When the Kundalini is awakened, the steps of Refining the Essence and Transforming the Qi happen by themselves. In fact, there is a limit to how much conscious effort you can put into Refining Essence and Transforming Qi. Of course, breathing can be used to refine essence and transform Qi, but it is not possible for a person to consciously breathe and observe 24 hours a day. As you develop yourself with these exercises, you move into a state where this development happens automatically.

When the process of Refining Essence and Transforming Qi begins to happen automatically, the progress of the training is much faster. Therefore, when the essence of life is generated in the body before it is consumed in any form, the process of Refining the Essence and Transforming Qi will automatically take place, and it will be transformed into Qi.

In the initial stages of Seon Do practice, the most important mantra is 'Eungshin-Ip-Qi-Hyeol' (凝神入氣穴), which is crucial for the automatic occurrence of the 'Yeon-Jeong-Hwa-Qi' (煉精化氣, Refining the Essence and Transforming Qi) process. 'Eungshin-Ip-Gi-Hyeol' translates as 'Focusing the Mind into the Qi Point', which means immersing the consciousness in the energy channels. This step is considered the first gate in Seon Do practice. It is the foundation for all subsequent practices, so its importance cannot be overstated. Although it is central, it is also beneficial to do it in parallel with breathing exercises. However, it is crucial to understand that 'Eungshin-Ip-Gi-Hyeol' (concentrating the spirit in the Qi point) takes precedence, with breathing following as a supporting practice.

When you breathe, the sensation of the perineum arises, which is the energy of the Lower Dantian, as if there were a pouch-like rubber ball in the lower abdomen, expanding and contracting with each breath. When the moonlight of consciousness shines on this, it is exactly as the scripture describes as if a clam opens its mouth to receive the moonlight and produces a pearl; a sari is produced from the pouch of the Qi cavities in the Lower Dantian.

This sari does not stay still but often begins to vibrate in an attempt to expand itself within the body. When this vibration begins, it is critical to swiftly use consciousness to guide it into the cavity of the coccyx. It then ascends along the spine, piercing through the nodes, going up to the back of the neck, passing through the medulla, and entering the skull. However, this is only possible when there is regular circulation through the conception and governor vessel, also known as the microcosmic orbit.

Governor vessel (督脈) commonly refers to the vessels flowing under the skin; indeed, all vessels of the body run just beneath the skin. However, once the sari is formed, it does not follow the typical path of the conception and governor vessel; instead, it follows its own route, which is referred to as the Route of Dan (丹道). The process of the sari circulating the front and back of the body along this path is called Dan Do Orbit (丹道周天). The energy cultivated through the Dan Orbit is immense, and the changes and phenomena are so different from person to person and so varied whenever they occur that it is impossible to describe them in words.

Of course, the Dan Do Orbit (丹道周天) is not something that can occur in everyone. If the state of Dan Orbit has been achieved, it would not be an exaggeration to say that the person has joined the ranks of immortals. In truth, when the circulation of the conception and governor vessels, known as the Microcosmic Orbit (Sojucheon), remains steady, the body will undergo a gradual Qi transformation.

The scriptures describe the ultimate state of this transformation as becoming a body without a shadow, which is indicative of a body that has undergone the process of Qi transformation (氣化). The legend of the immortals, or celestial beings (神仙), who sustain life solely on dew and heavenly Qi, directly points to this phenomenon.

When the body undergoes extreme Qi transformation, it reaches the stage of 'Leaving Earth and Becoming Immortal' (羽化登仙; a Daoist concept that describes the transformation and ascension of a person to become an immortal being.) Leaving Earth and Becoming Immortal refers to the body becoming so light that it can fly. Such entities can be frequently encountered not only in the Way of Immortals but also in the practices of Tantric yogis. Currently, only the tradition of Tibetan Buddhism maintains this lineage.

The traditions of Himalayan Yoga and Tantrism have all melted into one within Tibetan Buddhism. Also, in Indian Yoga, the lineage of Kundalini has been severed, as such traditions from the past could not be widely propagated among the masses. This is because the yogis of the snow mountains have become one with Tibetan Buddhism. Of course, now even Tibetan Buddhism is becoming secularized, so only the native Togal practitioners can make this possible, but their religious lineage has been cut off in secular terms.

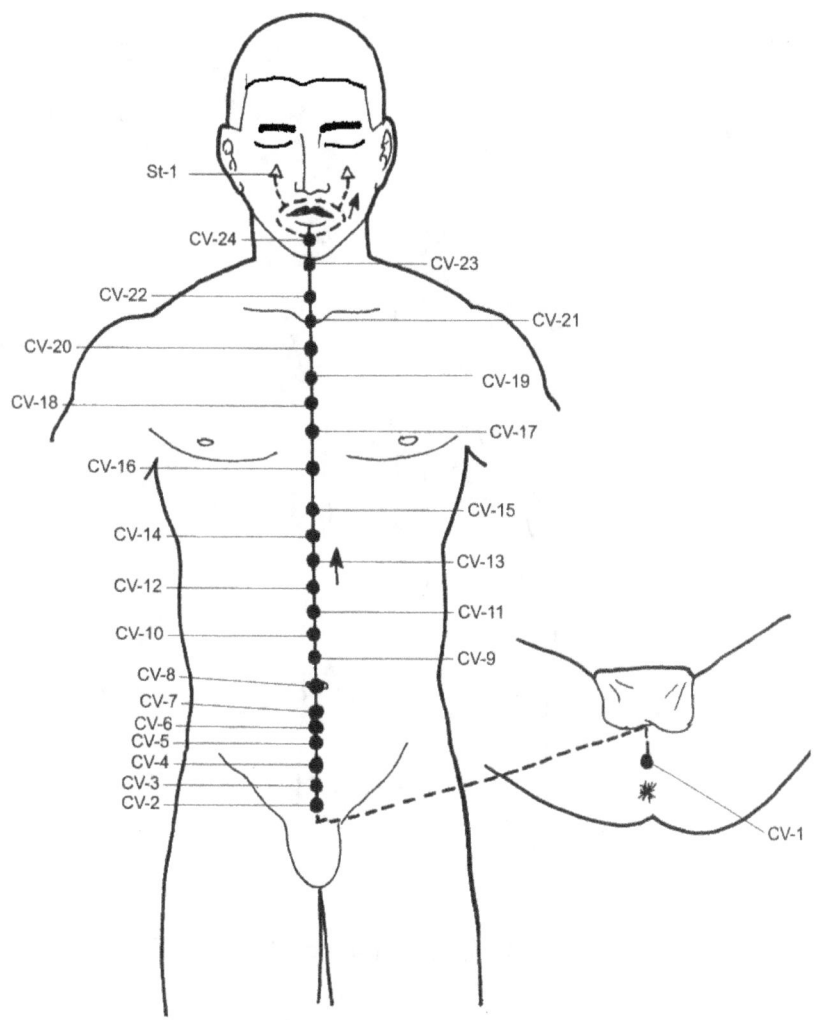

Conception Vessel (CV)

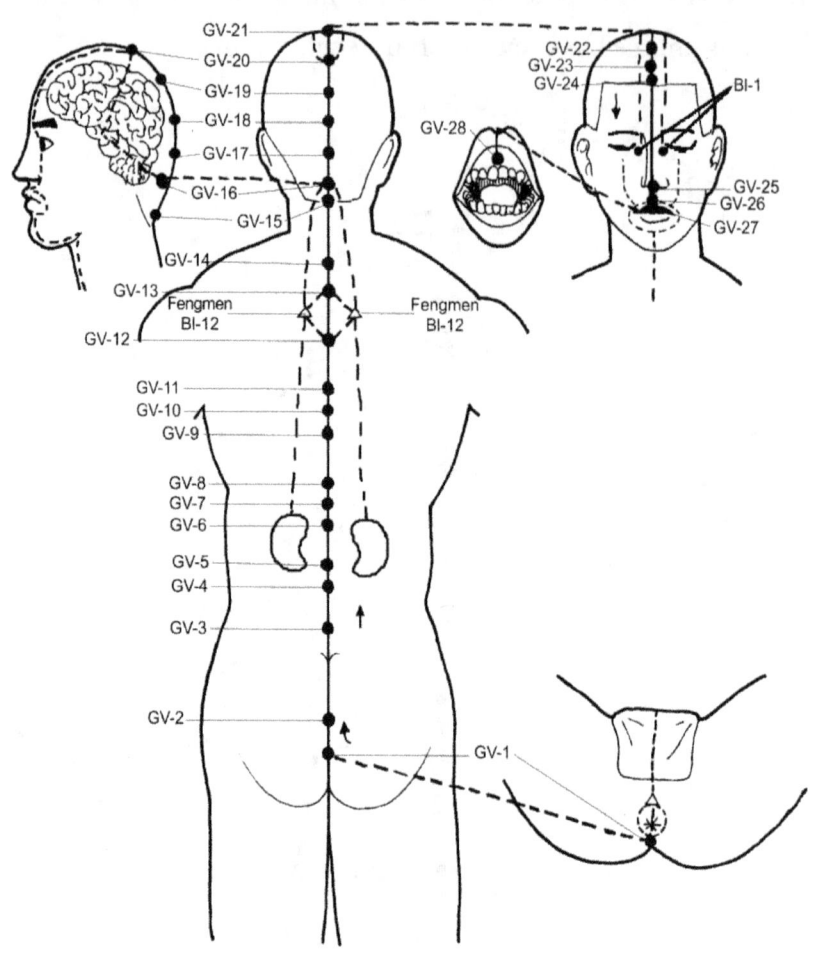

Governing Vessel (GV)

Chapter VIII. Breathing Techniques

Golden Rishi Qigong involves the entire process of Refining Essence and Transforming Qi (煉精化氣), Refining Qi and Transforming Spirit (鍊氣化神), and Cultivating the Spirit and Returning to Emptiness (鍊神還虛), all centered around seated meditation. Therefore, almost all stages utilize methods of meditation. While proper practice may take more time, here we introduce methods of meditation that can be practiced in a short time within the busy modern world to find stability in the body and mind.

A. Breathing Method to Clear the Mind (Upper Dantian Breathing)

By using hand seals as shown in Figures 1 and 2, receive the heavenly Qi into the GV20[83] (百會; Baeghoe) or the point between the eyebrows (印堂; EX-HN3) for about five minutes, eliminating distracting thoughts and awakening the palace of nirvana (泥丸宮). This helps to alleviate stress, the rising Qi disease, and neurotic disorders.

---

[83] Baeghoe is located on the top of the head, at the intersection of the midline and a line drawn between the apexes of the ears.

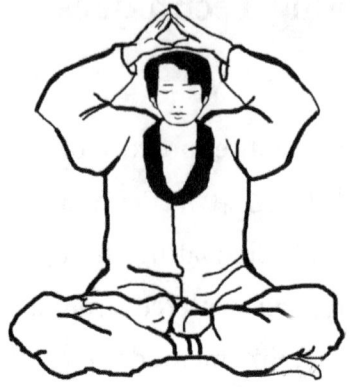
Figure 1

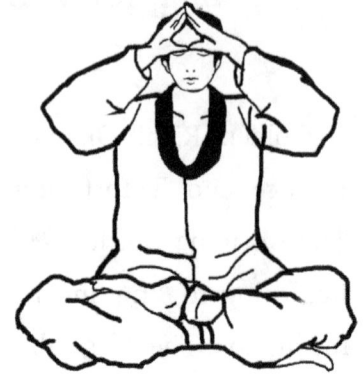
Figure 2

B. Breathing Method to Control the Mind (Middle Dantian Breathing)

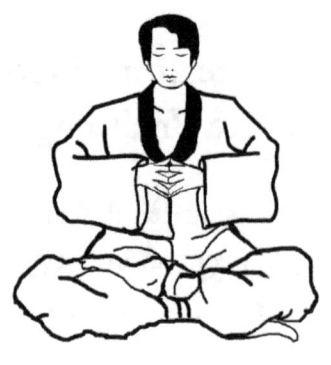
Figure 3

By using hand seals as shown in Figure 3, receive the human Qi into the CV12[84] (中脘; Zhongwan) acupoint for about five minutes, stabilizing the mind through the practices of cultivating (修心), illuminating (明心), and purifying (淨心) the mind. This helps to alleviate diseases such as heartburn and anger disorder.

---

[84]CV12 is located in the center of the abdomen, roughly four finger-widths above the navel.

C. Breathing Method to Control the Body's Equilibrium (Lower Dantian Breathing)

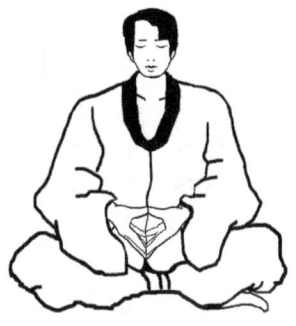

By using hand seals as shown in Figure 4, receive the earth Qi into the lower Dantian for about five minutes, gathering it in the lower Dantian to stabilize it. This helps to restore health and vitality.

Figure 4

D. Meditation Breathing Practice Method

If you have only a short time due to a busy daily schedule, here are some mindfulness practices to help you get in touch with your body and mind. First, relax the tension in your entire body and sit quietly with your mind collected and calm (收心靜坐).

Open the Heavenly Gate at GV20 (百會 Baeghoe ; crown). Through the GV20 (百會), receive the heavenly Qi and collect it at the point between the eyebrows, the tip of the nose, the front of the chest, and the Lower Dantian. Open the KD1[85] (涌泉; earthly gate) and draw up the earth Qi, collecting it in the KD1, the calves, the thighs and the

---

[85] sole of the foot

lower Dantian. Open the PC8⁸⁶ (勞宮, Laogong; the Human Gate), receive the Qi, and collect it in both arms, shoulders, CV22⁸⁷ (天突 Cheondol; the hollow at the base of the throat), chest, and lower Dantian. Prepare to exchange the vital energy of nature by opening all 84,000 pores of the body.

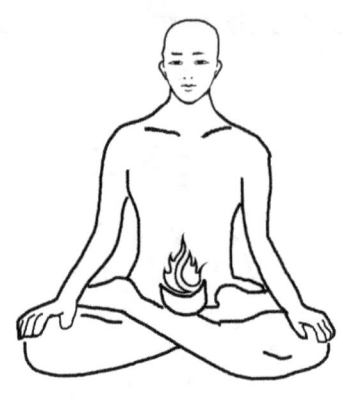

Open your eyes and gaze into the distance while projecting the divine light emanating from the Palace of Nirvana through the point between your eyebrows (印堂; EX-HN3). The farther you can look, the better. Gradually draw the transformed divine light back to your eyes and receive it at EX-HN3 (印堂; Third Eye). Gather your intention and gently lower it to the tip of your nose and then down to your heart. As your eyes gently close, turn your attention to the lower Dantian. Concentrate your intention on the lower Dantian. As you eliminate all distracting thoughts and concentrate on the lower Dantian, you enter a state of deep Samadhi.

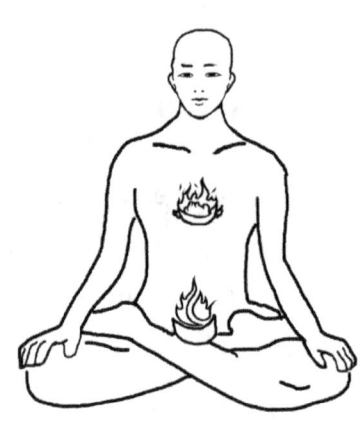

---

⁸⁶ palm of the hand
⁸⁷ on the midline of the throat

When the Qi accumulates in the lower Dantian and the energy becomes full, direct the energy of the lower Dantian to the middle Dantian. Concentrate your intention in the middle Dantian[88] and cultivate the mind through cultivation (修心), enlightenment (明心), and purification (淨心), and enter samadhi[89]. Reflect on your past self, free yourself from attachments, and evolve through the path of true reflection.

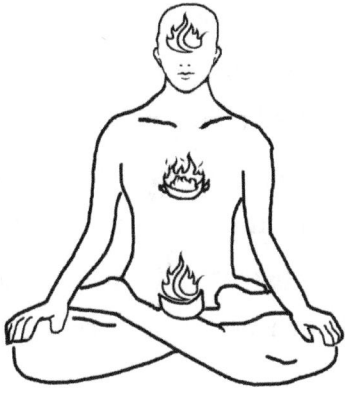

Then elevate the energy of the middle Dantian together with your intention to the upper Dantian and practice the cultivation of the Celestial Eye Point (天目穴 ; spiritual vision). First, focus your energy and intention on the Palace of Nirvana and enter samadhi to closely observe your present self. Then send your energy and intention to the post-heavenly mirror, concentrate, and enter samadhi to closely observe your past and previous life self[90]. Finally, turn your eyes forward, send your energy and intention,

---

[88] Cultivation in the Middle Dantian focuses on three key elements: refining the mind to achieve calmness and focus (Cultivation), gaining profound insight into one's existence (Enlightenment), and purging negative emotions and thoughts for a clearer state of mind (Purification). It's like tuning the mind, experiencing epiphanies, and cleansing the psyche to attain inner harmony.

[89] Samadhi: A state of meditative consciousness for the attainment of spiritual liberation, joyful calm, beyond absolute bliss.

[90] Observing the Past and Previous Life Self: What to notice: This step involves delving into your past, including the concept of past lives. The focus is on understanding how past experience have shaped your present self.

concentrate, and enter samadhi to observe your future and next-life self.

When you feel like you're waking up from samadhi and returning to reality, gather your intention in the lower Dantian and seal it in the lower Dantian to store the energy. Rub your palms together until they are hot, then place the warm energy of your palms over your eyes and infuse the warm energy deeply into your eyes. Then rotate your eyes three times to the left and three times to the right to finish. With this meditation method, the lower, middle, and upper Dantian can each be practiced for about 5 minutes or longer, depending on individual ability. It is suitable for busy modern people who can practice whenever they have a moment. In addition to the sitting position, it can also be practiced in the side-lying and supine positions.

Chapter IX. Golden Rishi Qigong

Through the basic Qi accumulation process of Golden Rishi Qigong, one can learn various practices such as performing Qi exercises, sleep meditation, wood meditation (exchanging Qi with trees), walking meditation (exchanging Qi with nature), sun meditation, and moon meditation. In addition, outdoor mountain training involves seeking mountains with abundant Qi and absorbing nature's vital energy to build up the body. After adjusting the body, breath, and mind through sitting methods and breathing techniques, the foundation is laid for circulating the Qi of the five elements in our bodies. This allows for the accumulation of Qi, thus laying the foundation for the circulation of the microcosmic orbit through Golden Rishi Qigong.

Earlier, we examined the interrelationships of the organs. As shown in the Five Elements Qi Diagram, Golden Rishi Qigong involves circulating Qi through the body's five major organs, considering their images and the theory of mutual nourishment and support of the five elements. Please see the directional lines on the diagram below to understand which organs support other organs. There are specific pathways. It is a practice method handed down from ancient times that serves as the foundation for internal cultivation. The method is recorded in the Diagram of Cultivating Truth (修眞圖), and it is used to nourish and treat each organ. It can also be used to treat others.

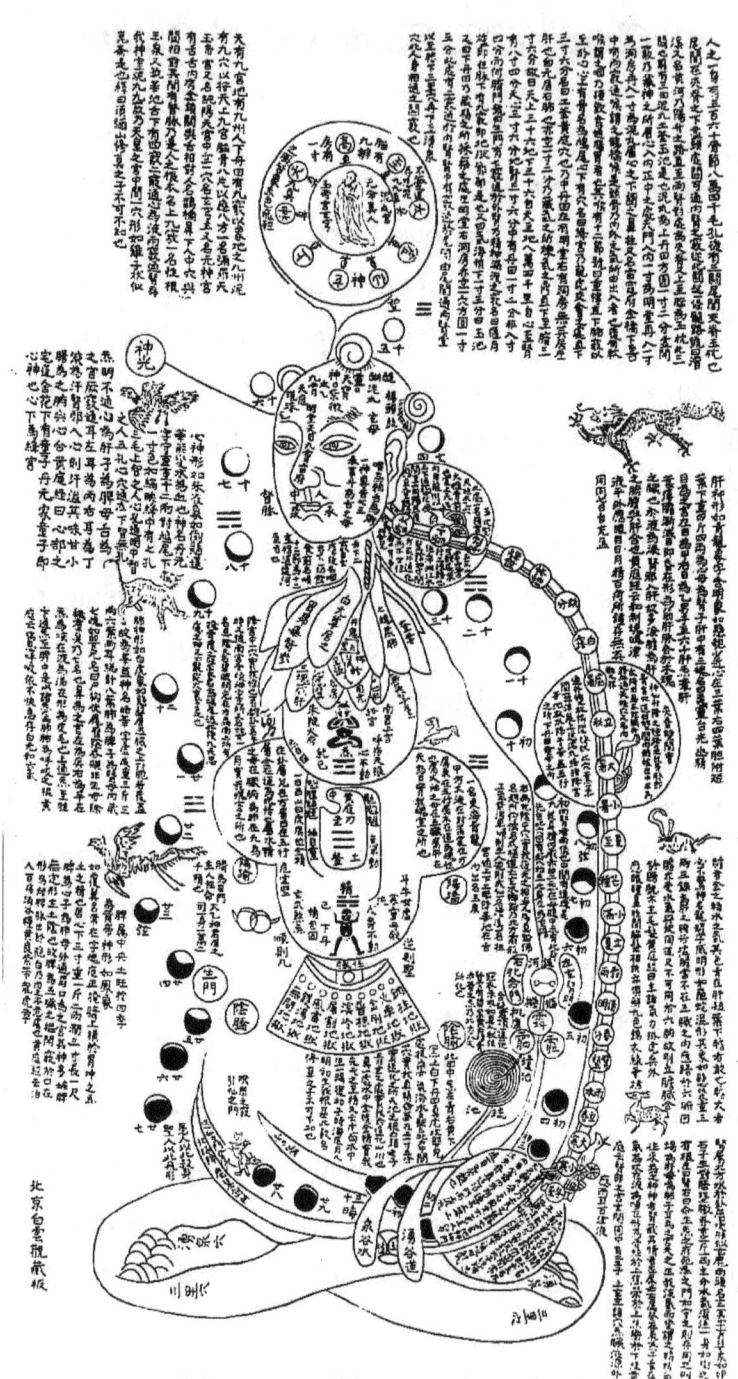

Diagram of Cultivating Truth

五行氣圖 (Five Elements Qi Diagram)

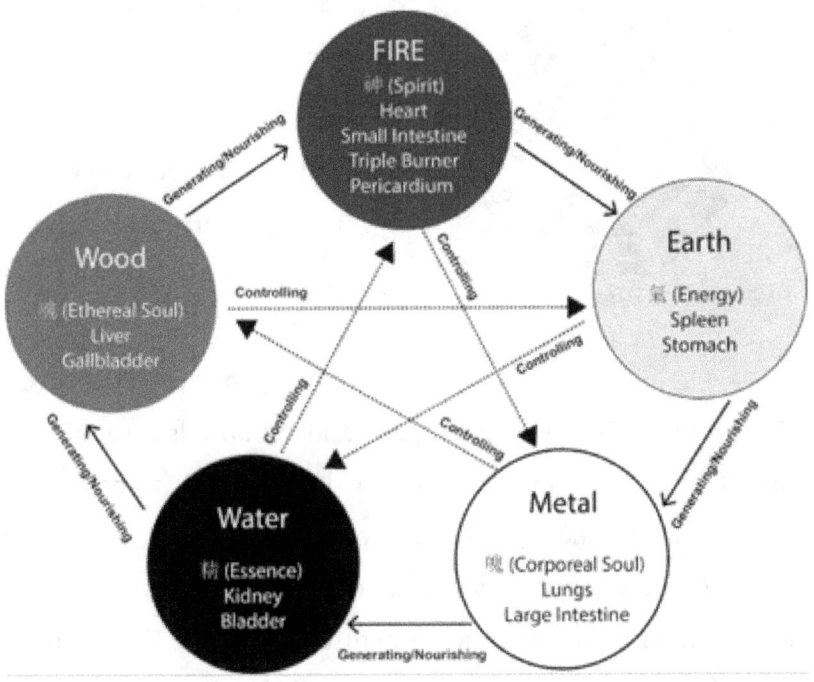

The secrets of the Taiji diagram (illustrating Yin and Yang) are also embedded in the five elements of Qigong. On the Five Elements Qi Diagram, the lines on the left and right, from the kidneys to the bladder, are the two aspects of Yin and Yang. After reaching the bladder, they merge into a single, rotating diagonal line that connects and reaches the liver and the heart. From the heart to the stomach and then to the lungs, another diagonal line is formed. In this way, a three-dimensional Taiji diagram is constructed. Within this diagram, there are two hidden openings that represent the fisheyes of Yin and Yang in the Taiji diagram.

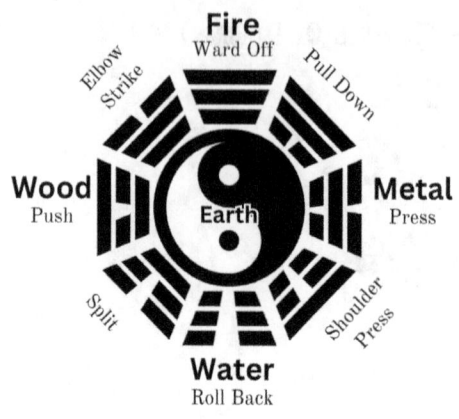

Master Zhong Yang (王重陽, 1112-1170 CE) called this the Little Return of the Elixir (小还丹), which is exactly the path of the Mao-You Orbit (卯酉周天) practice. When one reaches a certain level in the practice of the five elements of Qigong, one can transform the essence of life (精) in the five organs and six bowels into Qi in each organ. This begins the process of internal Qi transformation. Externally, when the Qi of the five organs is full, spontaneous movements occur, such as the hands lightly tapping along the meridian lines following the acupuncture points. The Qi liquefies and turns back into the elixir (丹), which is called the return of the elixir, meaning "to go out and return to the original place." The controlling relationship of the five elements was referred to in ancient times as "husband and wife using each other (夫妻盗用)," which is the intersection of metal and wood (金木交并), the combination of water and fire (水火相合), and also the harmonious coexistence of water and fire (水火濟濟).

The practice of Golden Rishi Five Elements Qigong consists of three stages:

- Stage 1: Use external Qi to push and circulate the Qi of the five organs.

- Stage 2: Use internal Qi to push and circulate the Qi of the five organs.
- Stage 3: Combine celestial and cosmic forces to push and circulate the Qi of the five organs.

Golden Rishi Five Elements Qigong is divided into two types: Single Form Qigong and Five Elements Qigong.

A. Golden Rishi Single-Form Qigong

This Qigong practice follows a route that operates independently based on the nourishment of the internal organs and the excretion pathways. The single route of Qigong can be divided into five types: kidney, liver and gallbladder, heart, stomach, and lungs. However, the kidney, liver, and gallbladder are combined and will be explained separately below.

To begin the practice, follow these steps:

Take off your glasses and watch, loosen your belt, and assume a half-lotus position. Relax your entire body, sit quietly with your eyes lowered and closed, roll your tongue up to touch the roof of your mouth, and meditate quietly while eliminating distracting thoughts.

Collect Qi in the lower Dantian through your breathing. From here, perform the single-form Qigong in the following order:

1. Stomach Qigong

Raise your hands and gather them under your chin with your palms facing down. Use the energy emanating from PC8 (勞宮 Nogung

; center of the palm) to press down along the esophagus. Visualize the size, shape, and color of your stomach. While stacking your hands in a hollow, cupped state, send energy between the cupped hands and stomach to nourish the stomach with Qi. Expel the toxin and send it down along the duodenum and small intestine. Continue to push the waste along the digestive tract, from the end of the small intestine to the ascending colon, transverse colon, descending colon, sigmoid colon, rectum, and finally to the anus, and expel the impurities. Then visualize and send away the forms of the organs that have been activated at a distance, observing them while practicing "Hwigwangbanjo" (回光返照) which means returning the light to illuminate within.

Stomach Qigong

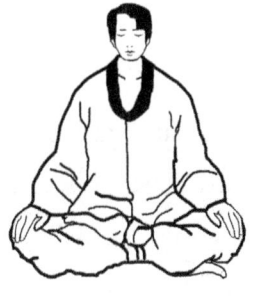

Stomach Qigong 1

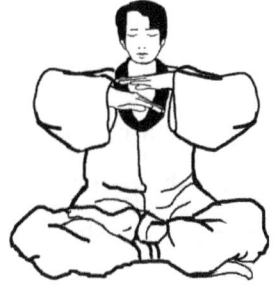

Stomach Qigong 2

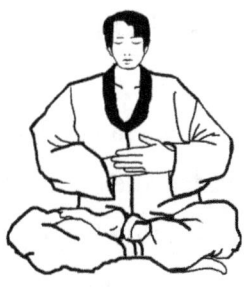

Stomach Qigong 3

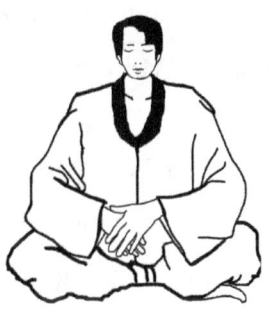

Stomach Qigong 4

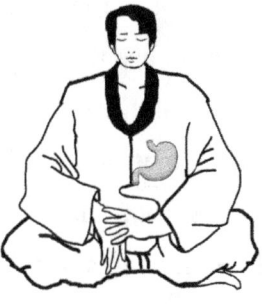

Stomach Qigong 5

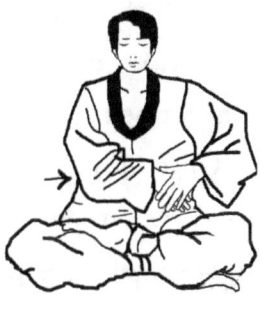

Stomach Qigong 6

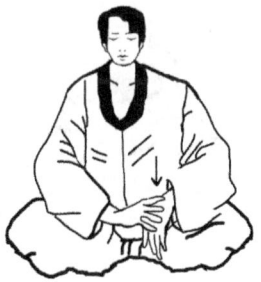

Stomach Qigong 7

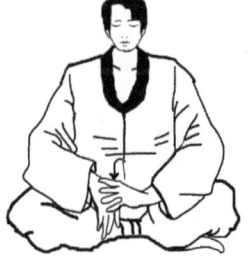

Stomach Qigong 8

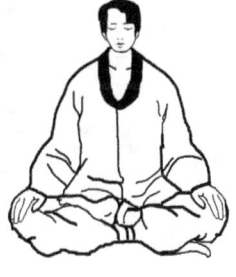

Stomach Qigong 9

2. Lung Qigong

In a seated meditation position, raise both hands and gather them under the chin, directing the palms downward. Use the energy emanating from the center of the palm (勞宮, Nogung) to push down along the bronchi.

At the point where the bronchi divide, separate your hands and, with the energy from your hands, thoroughly push and rotate the lung area, which spans from the ribs to the collarbone, in a state of vigorous activity. Simultaneously, visualize the shape, size, and color of the Qi-transformed lungs and nourish the lungs.

Once the energy transformation is sufficient, place both hands on your knees in a peaceful position. Throw the image of the lung area far away and observe it while drawing and reflecting the returning light.

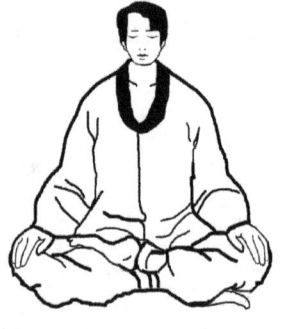

Lung Qigong 1

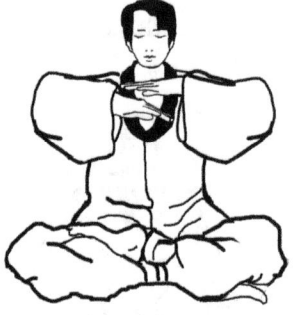

Lung Qigong 2

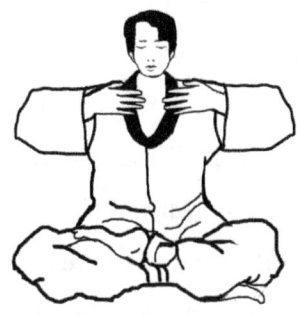 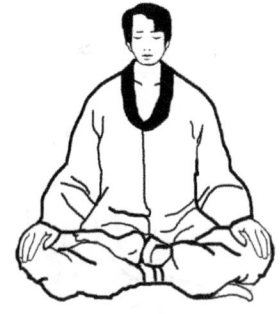

Lung Qigong 3   Lung Qigong 4

3. Kidney and Liver Qigong

In the seated meditation posture, with your eyes closed, extend your gaze far and collect the 'shingwang' (divine light) energy between your eyebrows. Channel this energy in the order of the Qi Cavity (穴), the Upper Dantian (目), and the Third Eye (天; Mirror), and let it descend along the spine until it reaches the kidneys. While maintaining a certain distance (隔空; "gekgong" or "separated space"), use both hands to energetically circulate and enliven the kidneys. At the same time, visualize the energized state of the kidneys by observing their size, shape, and color. This process is about nourishing and revitalizing the kidneys through the circulation of Qi (炁), ensuring that they are well supported and energized. Push the Qi from both kidneys along the urethral canal toward the bladder. Observe and visualize the size,

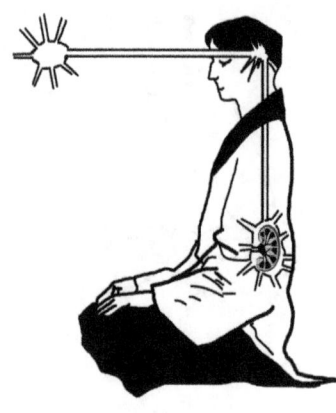

shape, and color of the bladder with your hands clasped together while carefully circulating the energy.

Then direct the Qi from the bladder up toward the liver. With the hands still overlapped, carefully circulate and invigorate the liver, observing the color, size, and shape of the energized liver, thereby nourishing and revitalizing it (補氣). By carefully pressing and guiding the energy through the gallbladder and following the bile ducts to the liver, one can expel toxins (濁氣) from the liver. This is done by methodically pushing the turbid Qi through the digestive tract, starting from the duodenum, through the small intestine, ascending colon, transverse colon, descending colon, sigmoid colon, rectum, and finally the anus. In a quiet sitting posture (靜坐), with the hands on the knees and the eyes closed, one visualizes looking far away to the horizon. This visualization involves sending the images of the energized organs far away for observation, a process known as "returning the light to illuminate within" (廻光返照).

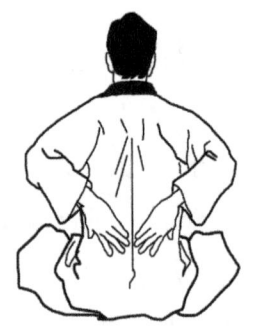

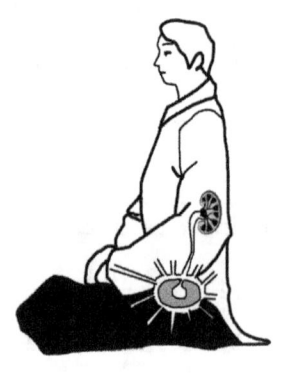

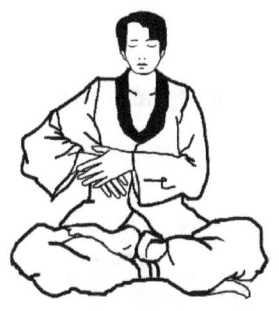
Liver Qigong 1

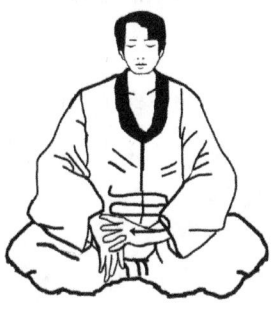
Liver Qigong 2

Liver Qigong 3

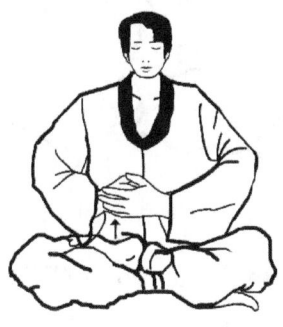
Liver Qigong 4

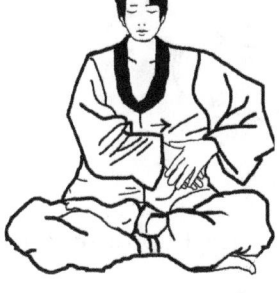
Liver Qigong 5

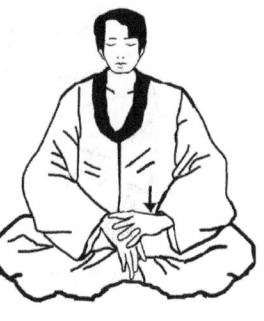
Liver Qigong 6

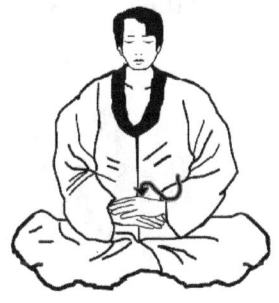
Liver Qigong 7

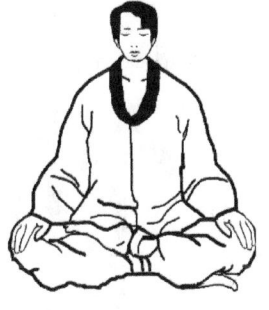
Liver Qigong 8

4. Heart Qigong

In a seated meditation position, raise both hands and circulate around the heart while visualizing the shape, color, and size of the heart.

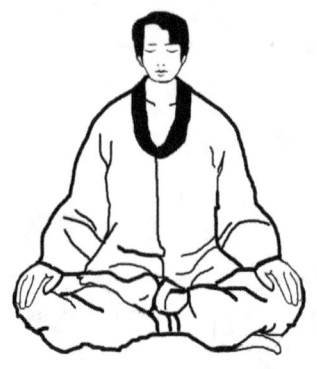
Heart Qigong 1

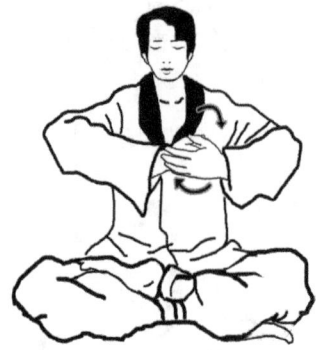
Heart Qigong 1

Lift the Qi (炁) of the heart upwards, and from the acupoint CV22 (天突,) Chundol, the center point where the collarbone meets, move it towards both shoulders. From the shoulders, direct it to the elbows, from the elbows to the wrists, and finally to the tips of the fingers. As you exhale, push out the turbid energy.

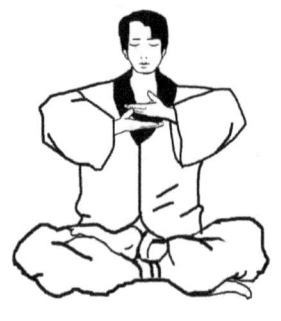
Heart Qigong 3

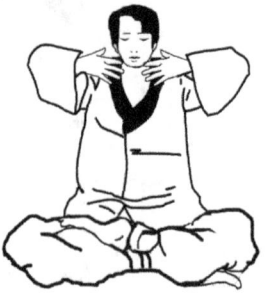
Heart Qigong 4

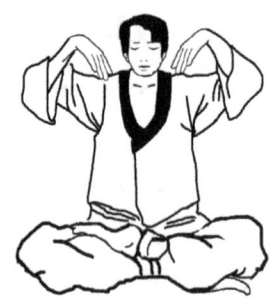
Heart Qigong 5

As you inhale, draw the heavenly Qi from the fingertips to the wrists, from the wrists to the elbows, from the elbows to the shoulders, from the shoulders to the CV22 (天突), and then to the heart. This process cleanses the ascending aorta and vena cava, efficiently converting and conveying the energy of the heart.

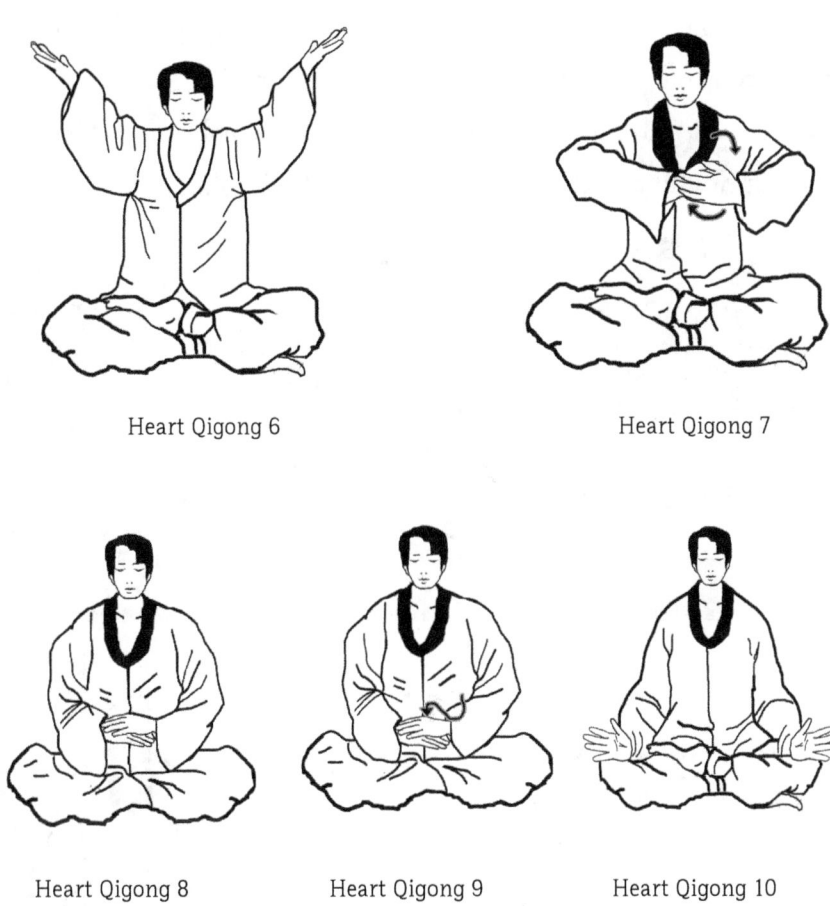

Heart Qigong 6 Heart Qigong 7

Heart Qigong 8 Heart Qigong 9 Heart Qigong 10

Push the Qi (炁) of the heart downwards to the Lower Dantian, and as you exhale, divide the energy from the Lower Dantian towards both sides, continuing through the thighs, calves, ankles, and to the tips of the toes, expelling the turbid energy.

Then, as you inhale, gather energy in the reverse order, that is, from the tips of the toes, ankles, calves, and thighs, up to the Lower Dantian, and finally to the heart. This process purifies the descending aorta and the vena cava and once again effectively transforms and transports the energy of the heart.

Send the visualized shape of the manipulated organ into the distance while naturally placing your hands on your knees. With your eyes closed, carefully observe the shape that has been sent afar, and then draw and reflect the returning light (廻光返照).

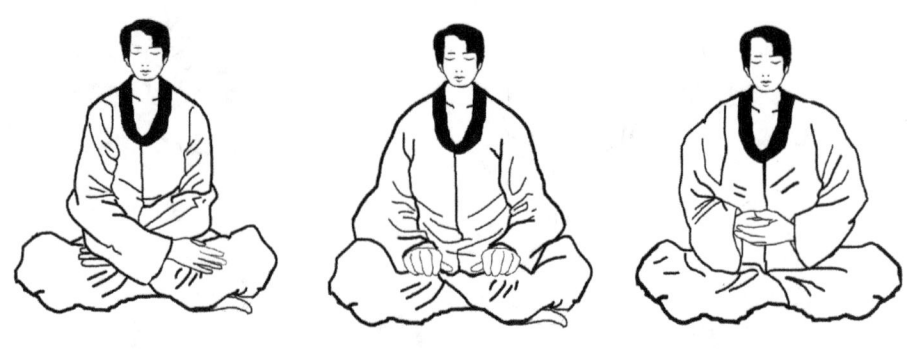

Heart Qigong 11 Heart Qigong 12 Heart Qigong 13

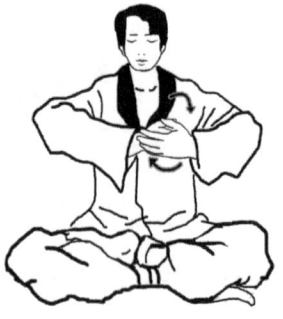 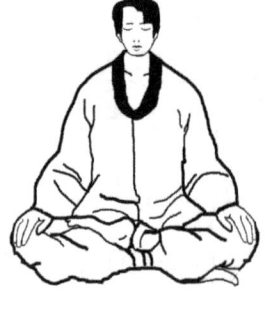

Heart Qigong 14 Heart Qigong 15

B. Golden Rishi Five Elements Qigong

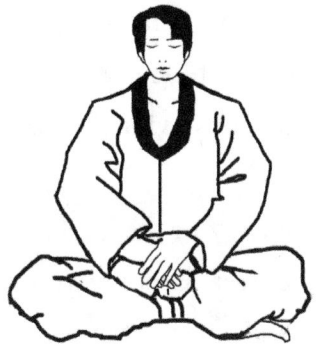

1) Take off your eyeglasses and wristwatch and loosen your belt to adopt a half lotus position (or a natural seated position). Relax your entire body and sit still. Lower your eyes and gently close them, curl your tongue to touch the roof of your mouth, and quietly meditate while clearing away distracting thoughts.

2) Gather energy in the Lower Dantian through your breath.

3) Place your hands overlapping on the Lower Dantian and rotate the energy from your palms clockwise to cultivate[91] the energy in the Lower Dantian.

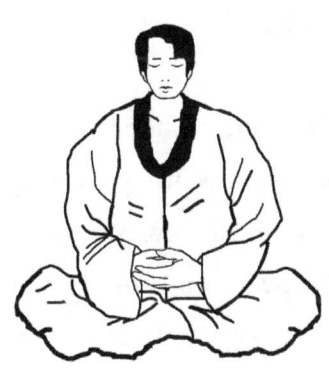

4) As you inhale, pull out the Refining Lifeline (壽命綫)[92], and as you exhale, return the Lifeline to its original position. Observe whether the coccyx moves along and feels stimulated as you repeat this several times. Again, rotate the hands clockwise around the Lower Dantian with the overlapping hands.

---

[91] How to Cultivate Qi: practice slow, deep breathing while focusing on the Lower Dantian, drawing energy to this center with each breath and sensing warmth or vibrations.

[92] Refining Lifeline involves cultivating energy along the pathway from the Dantian (丹田) to the Milyeo (尾閭) to enhance longevity and overall vitality.

5) Bring the energy from the Lower Dantian down to the bladder with both hands. With your eyes closed, focus all your intent and gaze on the bladder, and circulate the bladder's energy with the energy from both hands. Gently rotate and cultivate the bladder, observing its size, color, shape, and the substances inside.

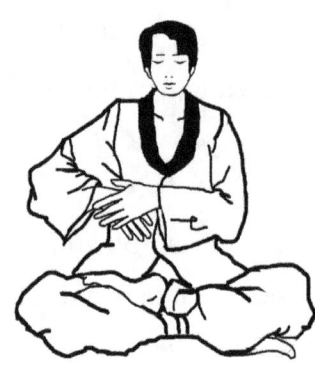

6) Gather the energy in the bladder and bring it to the liver. Keeping your eyes closed, focus all your intent and gaze on the liver, and circulate the liver's energy with the energy from both hands. While earnestly raising and transforming the liver's energy with both hands, observe the cultivated liver's size, color, and shape, and continue to cultivate while sensing the reaction that appears in the eyes, which are the sensory openings (明竅) of the liver.

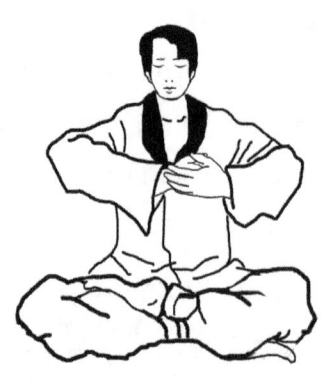

7) Collect the energy of the liver and bring it to the heart. With your eyes closed, concentrate all your thoughts and gaze on the heart, and rotate your heart with the energy of your hands. Continue to cultivate the heart with the energy of both hands, carefully observing the size, color, and shape of the cultivated heart and feeling the tongue's response to the sensory openings of the heart.

8) Gather the heart's energy and bring it down to the spleen. With your eyes closed, focus all your thoughts and gaze on the spleen, and rotate the spleen's energy with the energy from your hands. Observe the size, color, and shape of the cultivated spleen. Feel the reaction that appears in the mouth and limbs, which are the sensory openings (明竅) of the spleen, as you continue to cultivate the energy and attention from your hands.

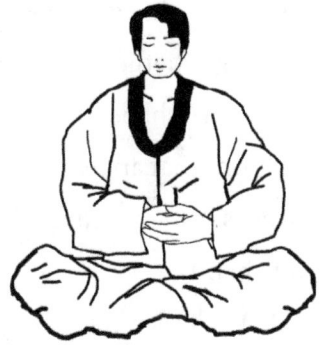

9) Gather the energy from the spleen and stomach and spread it to both lungs with your hands. With

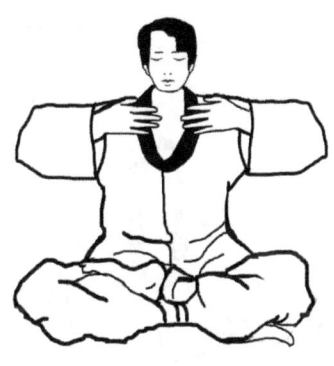

your eyes closed, concentrate on all your thoughts and focus on your lungs. Turn and transform the lungs with the energy of your hands.

As you carefully rotate the lungs with the energy from your hands and transform them with Qi, observe the size, color, and shape of the lungs. Check whether both lungs are the same size. Pay attention to the reaction in the nose, which is the bright opening (明竅) of the lungs, while carefully transforming the lungs with the energy from your hands.

10) Gather the energy from both lungs and bring it along the ribs to the bilateral kidneys. With your eyes closed, focus all your thoughts and attention on the kidneys. Use the energy from your hands to rotate and cultivate the kidneys. Observe the size, color, and shape of the cultivated kidneys, noticing whether or not they are the same size and shape. Pay attention to any 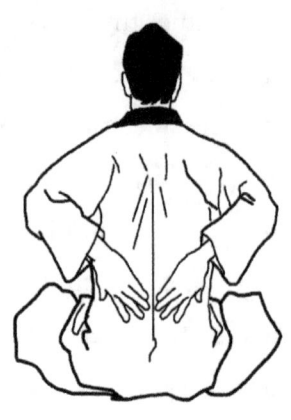 reactions that appear in the ears, which are the sensory openings of the kidneys, as you diligently cultivate the energy using the energy from your hands.

11) Gather the energy of the bilateral kidneys and bring it along the urethral canal to the bladder. With your eyes closed, concentrate all your thoughts and gaze on the bladder. Use the energy from both hands to rotate and diligently cultivate the bladder's energy. While carefully observing the size, color, and shape of the 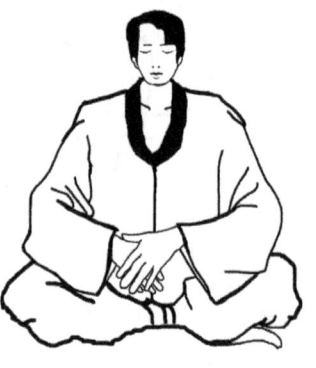 bladder, pay close attention to how the color has changed from before to after cultivation. Feel and experience the transformation.

12) After circulating through the bladder, circulate the energy in the following order: liver, heart, stomach, lungs, bilateral kidneys, and back to the bladder, creating an ascending action of the Five Elements. Repeat this circulation for three or six cycles before returning to the bladder.

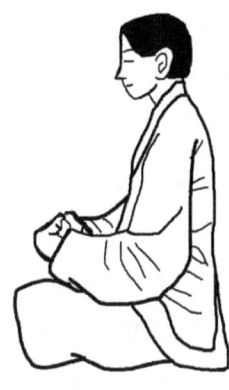

13) Gather the bladder's energy and bring it up to the Lower Dantian. With your eyes closed, focus all your thoughts and gaze on the Lower Dantian, and use the energy from both hands to rotate and diligently cultivate the energy of the Lower Dantian. First, feel and experience how the Lower Dantian has changed from before to after cultivation, and then continue to diligently cultivate the Lower Dantian using the energy from both hands.

14) While inhaling, pull in the Refining Lifeline from the Lower Dantian. Then, while exhaling, return the Lifeline to its original position, repeatedly performing the movement where the tailbone moves along and feels stimulated. Return to using the overlapping hands to rotate the Lower Dantian around in a clockwise fashion.

15) In front of the Lower Dantian, join your hands with your fingertips facing forward, raise your hands up to the chest area to the Middle Dantian while pointing your fingertips upward. Next, point your fingertips forward towards the horizon, while performing the Pulling of the Line of Strength out away from the torso. As you inhale, observe whether you can feel the EX-B2 (acupoints along the vertebra, 夾脊) being pulled while you pull forward with your hands together. As you exhale, return the Lifeline to its position inside the chest area. Repeat this several times within the body to provide sufficient stimulation to the EX-B2 (夾脊).

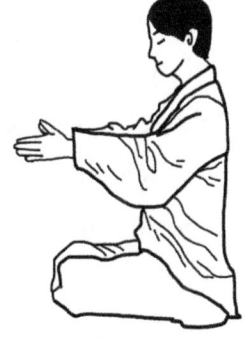

16) Place both hands on your knees with fingers spread apart and be still. Prepare for the microcosmic orbit explained next.

C. Sojucheon (小周天; The Microcosmic Orbit)

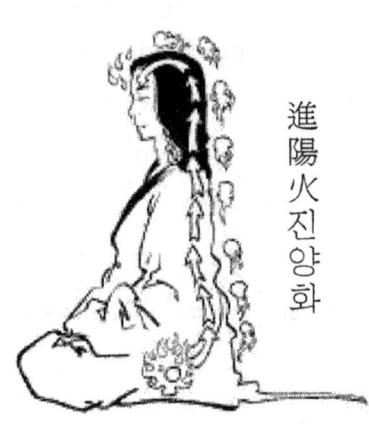

Through the Golden Rishi Qigong teaching, one learns various training methods of Qi accumulation including conducting Qi exercises (guided physical exercises), sleep meditation, the practice of wood meditation (exchanging Qi with trees), walking meditation (exchanging Qi with nature), sun meditation, and moon meditation.

After internalizing these methods, practitioners engage in outdoor mountain training and seek out mountains with abundant Qi. The practitioner absorbs nature's Qi to strengthen their bodies, refine the body, and cultivate Qi. Only after completing this process do they move on to Refining Essence and Transforming Qi.

Golden Rishi Academy in Korea extensively documents this part in the Methods of the Sacred Jewel (靈寶畢法) (2000.) However, beginners should start with the basics under the guidance of a competent teacher to ensure correct and efficient practice without trial and error.

The process of collecting energy, or storing Qi in the lower Dantian, and refining it is part of the practice. This involves focusing and heating the consciousness so that the essence of life is cultivated into Qi (炁), which can be intensely felt as heat.

Once the Qi (炁) is full, exhaling allows the Qi (炁) to flow down toward the CV1 (the area between the anus and the genitals; 會陰). As this happens, the Qi transforms into yang-in-yin (陰中陽), and the hot energy rises from the end of the coccyx, passes through the base of the spine (尾閭關), and ascends along the governor vessel (back side of torso) to the top of the head.

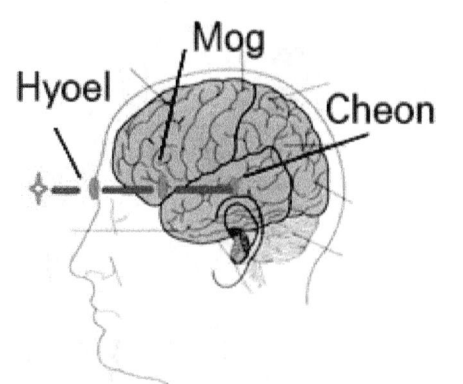

This process of channeling Qi along the governing vessel is known as advancing yang fire (進陽火), which indicates the upward movement of yang energy, or vital heat, within the body.

When this Qi reaches the Palace of Mog (see diagram), the pure yang Qi begins to transform into pure yin Qi, at which point cooling begins. Inhaling and allowing this cooled energy to reach from the Palace of Mog to the root of the earth, the cooled Qi flows from the EX-HN3 (印堂, Hyoel; forehead between brows), transferring Qi from EX-HN3 through the

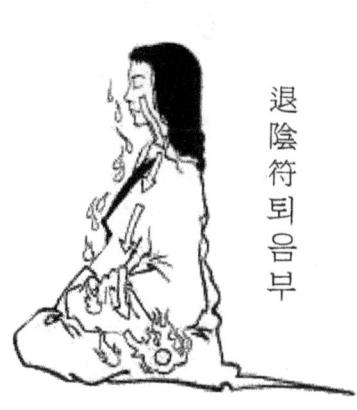

conception vessel to the Lower Dantian. This process (called 退陰符, or Tuiyinbu) describes the descent of cooled Qi back to the Lower Dantian through the conception vessel.

After guiding the Qi through the conception vessel and the governing vessel, it is important to stabilize the temperature and consistently practice the Sojucheon (Microcosmic Orbit) to enhance the essence in the Dantian. Only after this process is completed can one obtain the elixir (內丹).

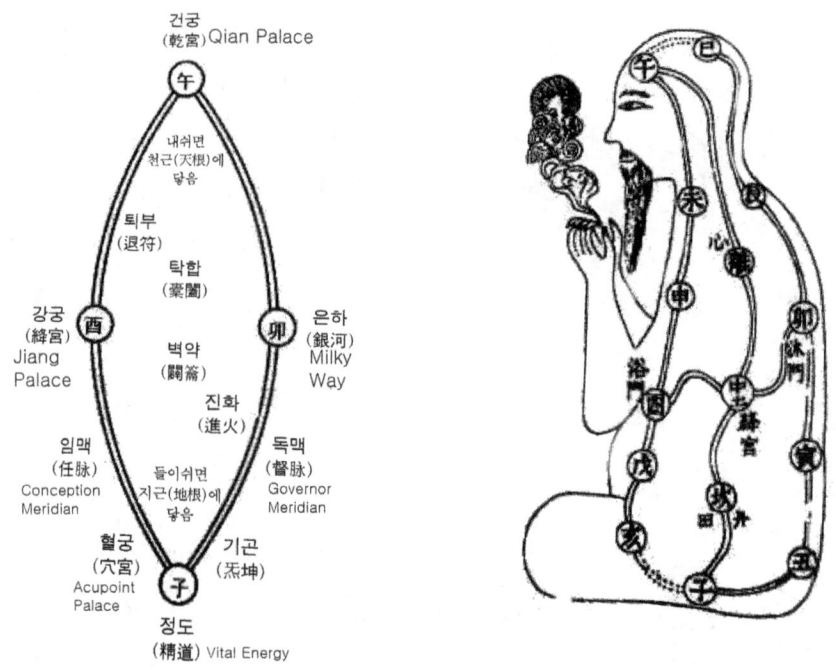

The harmonious rotation of the six energies according to the law.

It is important to penetrate any blockages and circulate through the conception and governing vessels. In this process, it is necessary to stabilize and circulate the Attainment of Heat (火候) as efficiently as possible, but how can we do that?

Heat attainment (火候) is the collective term in cultivation for intention, breathing, time, and method. The intention is fire, the breath is the wind, and the temperature encapsulates time and space. The fire is the intention, and it is the spirit, which is divided into yang fire and yin fire, yang and yin spirit. It involves inspiration and perceptions, among other phenomena, and is combined with breath in the practice.

In the fourth stage of breathing, after all the breath has been exhaled, the perineum is pulled up, and this pull ascends along the spine to GV20 (top of the head), where one finally inhales. Along with the inhalation, the consciousness flows under the skin in front of the neck through the conception vessel and collects in the perineum.

When exhaling, the Qi that has gathered in the pouch of the perineum is squeezed out, and the pelvic floor muscles are contracted at this time. After fully exhaling, one stops breathing, and the Qi ascends to the GV20 (top of the head), just like blocking the entrance of a syringe and laboriously lifting the cylinder to create a vacuum. This can be described as the unblocking method of the conception and governor vessel in respiration, which is to break through what is blocked.

What we need to pay attention to here is that if beginners who are over the age of 40 (unlike those in their 20s who are rich in the essence of life) start the breathing method to break through what has blocked the conception and governor vessels, they will experience the side effects of headaches. This condition is often termed Rising-Qi Disease

(上氣病), but it fundamentally differs from a headache caused by Qi rising along the conception vessel at the front of the body. This point must be clearly understood.

In most cases, those suffering from Rising-Qi Disease have experienced Qi rising along the conception vessel. As mentioned, this is due to excessive breath holding after inhaling, causing the Qi to reverse. In cases where pure Qi ascension occurs, i.e., Qi rises through the governor vessel to the top of the head, causing a headache, the flow of Qi is weak and cannot properly condense at the head due to high pressure, and it doesn't have the strength to descend. In this situation, the Qi stays in the head, causing a headache.

Such headaches occur because the process of Refining Essence and Transforming Qi is actively happening, and the essence of life is all being cultivated, so it can be thought of as the body's self-defense mechanism asking for new food and resting quickly. At that time, one should promptly consume protein-rich food, break from practice, and get sufficient rest. Once a certain amount of the essence of life is regenerated, the headache symptoms can be alleviated.

This process is essentially a step that everyone will likely go through. It is important to understand that it is not a side effect but a natural symptom and to respond wisely.

If the headache does not improve, the conception vessel might have been blocked while the governor vessel was opened. In that case, it is necessary to perform practice to unblock the conception vessel for a while. The practice to unblock the conception vessel is to visualize the Qi gathering in your head while you inhale, and then visualize it flowing down along the front of the body into the Qi cavities in the Lower Dantian.

At first, this may not work well, but after practice, it is as if the Qi cavity becomes a vacuum-like rubber ball and inflates, sucking in the Qi. The phenomenon occurs when the liquid of the flowing Qi rapidly flows down along the abdomen. It feels like a stream of water is flowing, or, to exaggerate a bit, the liquid of the Qi is flowing like a river.

If the conception vessel has not properly broken through what has been blocked, you may feel like the liquid is flowing down the surface of your face from your forehead. It continues down your entire face to your neck but doesn't go down any further and disperses. When this happens, your facial skin becomes very radiant and milky, producing a lot of oil and making it look as if you intentionally applied oil.

So, how should one deal with the Rising Qi Disease which occurs due to reverse flow? It is simple. Practice the four-stage breathing we have discussed here while performing the technique to unblock the conception and governor vessels. The basis for all these techniques is to 'concentrate the spirit to enter the Qi cavity.' One should actually feel as if there is a pouch in their Lower Dantian. Developing a strong awareness of this pouch and how energy moves in and out of it will be important to practice because various applications and advancements are derived from the sensation of this pouch.

The consciousness shall then be placed into the pouch. Just as placing a hot stone in cold water makes the water boil, inserting the conscious spirit (離火) into the Qi cavities of the Lower Dantian makes the essence boil. The conscious spirit refers to the fire of consciousness and is associated with the Li (離) trigram in the Book of

Changes (易經 [93]), which contains a yin in the middle and yang lines above and below, symbolizing a pot of boiling water, an analogy for consciousness.

Li(離)-Fire : is related to the Heart

Kan(坎) - Water : is related to the Kidneys

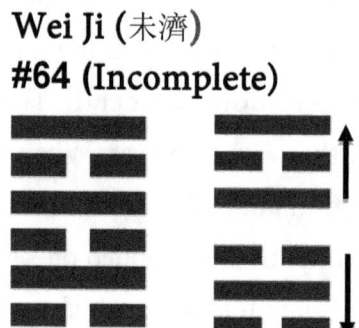

Wei Ji (未濟)
#64 (Incomplete)

Fire typically rises to the chest as light, while water descends to the Dantian due to its heaviness, representing the "post-heaven" or "after-birth" state. Hexagram #64 symbolizes the lack of integration and harmony, with fire positioned above and water below, moving in opposite directions, depicting a state of Not Yet Fulfilled or Incomplete.

Fire and water can create refined energy through steam and condensation, similar to heating water on a stove. This interaction requires balance, as excessive heat can cause water to evaporate, and overflowing water can extinguish the fire. This balance is represented by hexagram #63: Ji Ji (Completion), which shows the water trigram above the fire trigram, promoting mutual interaction and transformation between the two elements.

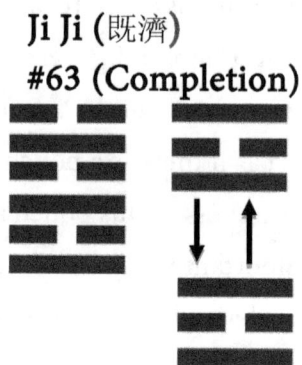

Ji Ji (既濟)
#63 (Completion)

---

[93] 易經 (Yì Jīng), often translated as the Book of Changes or I Ching, is one of the oldest Chinese classic texts. It is a foundational work in Chinese philosophy, cosmology, and divination.

Tai (夬) #11 (Peace)

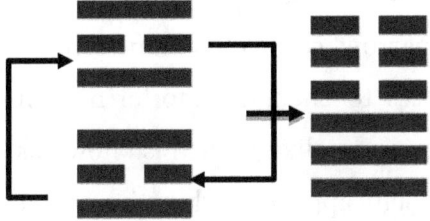

Through proper posture, breath control, and mental calmness, Dantian acts like a stove, transforming water into vapor that rises to the chest and heart, coalesces, and descends back to Dantian. In Daoist meditation, inner alchemy shifts the trigrams, creating Qian-Heaven and Kun-Earth, symbolized by Hexagram #11: Peace, representing a return to the pre-heaven state and reflecting Daoism's beliefs in halting temporal movement for "immortality" or practical peace and tranquility.

In contrast, the Kan (坎) trigram has a yang line in the middle and yin lines above and below, symbolizing water containing fire and referring to the essence produced by the energy of the kidneys. The basic principle of Seon Do, Refining Essence and Transforming Qi, involves not expelling this essence, but boiling it to transform it into Qi.

If one does not consciously focus breathing in a state of 'concentrating the spirit and entering the Qi cavity' (凝神入氣穴), the practice becomes pointless; it does not work. On the contrary, if one does not let go of the very end of one's breath, but keeps observing it, they will reach an intermediate state that is neither sleep nor fully awake and conscious. This state is referred to in ancient scriptures as 'neither forgetting nor assisting' (勿忘勿助), a metaphor for the state of meditation. In other words, if one doesn't fall into unconsciousness or enter the current consciousness, but stands on the boundary of both sides, a moment of transcendence occurs. This process is half the study of Refining Essence and Transforming Qi (煉精化氣).

The remaining half involves the cultivated essence coalescing into a form that permeates all the bone marrow, completely transforming one's constitution. This process refers to changing mortal human bones into spiritual bones by consuming an elixir, which is known as the Golden Elixir. At this point, a sign appears within the Lower Dantian, specifically the emergence of a small, shining bead. This bead is considered the true seed, also known as the seed of elixir.

When one emerges from deep meditation or deep sleep, one can experience the awakening hour state. This happens because the kidney water (腎水 or 坎水), or the fluid of the kidneys, is drawn up by the fire of consciousness (神火 or 離火) and gathered by the Qi cavity (氣穴; energy point) of the Lower Dantian. The reason to concentrate on the Lower Dantian without allowing the fire of consciousness to ascend is to gather the kidney water and convert it into essence. This essence, in turn, when combined with the Qi of respiration, forms the seeds of elixir. Once this seed is obtained, its effect persists for as long as the body exists. Ultimately, even after the body is cremated, this seed remains in the form of a relic (small stone-like calcified relic).

Upon obtaining the seed of elixer, or sari, one's body becomes light and gentle, circulation throughout the hundred vessels becomes smooth, all diseases disappear, and longevity can be attained. Furthermore, if one studies deeply, it becomes a gateway to entering Samadhi and serves as the energy of meditation. Therefore, there is no longer a shortage of the original Qi, and all bodily discomfort is eliminated.

When in the awakening hour state, the practitioner should not hesitate, but use four methods simultaneously: Inhale (吸), Polish (砥), Grasp (撮), and Close(閉) the Qi of the spiritual seed, drawing it into the Qi cavity of the lower Dantian. When there, the practitioner should circulate it once through the microcosmic orbit, return it to the Qi cavity of the lower Dantian, and seal it there. This is the method of harvesting the elixir.

Inhale (吸) means to gather energy into the perineum; Polish (砥) means to place the tongue on the roof of the mouth; Grasp (撮) refers to tightening the anus; and Close(閉) means to close the eyes, ears, and mouth to concentrate. Harvest the elixir according to these four methods. If one continuously applies this fourfold technique to harvest the elixir, a vibration will occur in the Qi cavities of the Lower Dantian, and the gate of the Qi cavity will open. Then it feels as if breathing suddenly stops, and a bead appears like a single white grain is emerging in the darkness. Even now, one should use the four methods (四口訣) to harvest it. Then, this bead gradually solidifies and becomes what is called the Small Elixir. If this Small Elixir circulates the Sojucheon (Microcosmic Orbit) about 300 times through the path of the Conception and Governor Vessels, it turns into a golden Great Elixir called Dan (丹).

Eventually, these beads become the ingredients for the Great Elixir (大丹). Once this Great Elixir matures to a certain point, it rises, penetrating the barrier of the spine and reaching the brain. This stage represents the pinnacle of Sojucheon awakening and is the flower of Seon Do practice. Once the Great Elixir reaches the brain, one experiences enlightenment. After this, it descends to the Lower Dantian to be stored signifying the completion of the second stage: Refining Essence and Transforming Qi. Those who have completed this stage have been referred to as human immortals, adepts and sages. They have achieved the state of realization. One becomes a human immortal, one enjoys freedom from illness and aging throughout their life, enjoys longevity, and the body and face transform to radiate vitality and youthfulness. This is truly a 'Return to Youth from Old Age.'

The content of this book is intended to help one get started on their path of ultimate health. One should expect the study process to occur over many years of time. Dedicated, ongoing practice is the key to grasping understanding; insight occurs through individual enlightenment. Enlightenment happens when and as a person is ready for it.

Descriptions of Different Types of "Jucheon" (周天; orbits) Practices

1. **So Jucheon** (小周天; Microcosmic Orbit):
    - **Pathway**: Involves the Ren Meridian (任脈, CV) and the Du Meridian (督脈, GV). Qi starts from the Lower Dantian, travels up the Du Meridian along the spine, over the head, and down the Ren Meridian back to the Lower Dantian.

- **Features**: This fundamental practice balances and maintains internal Qi circulation, promoting overall health and equilibrium.
2. **Kan Li Jucheon (坎離周天; Water and Fire Orbit)**:
    - **Pathway**: Involves circulating Qi between the symbolic interactions of Water (Kan, ☵) and Fire (Li, ☲).
    - **Features**: Focuses on balancing the heart (fire) and the kidneys (water), fostering mental stability and harmony between mind and body.
3. **Zha Wu Jucheon (子午周天; Midnight and Noon Orbit)**:
    - **Pathway**: Practiced according to the time periods of Zha (midnight) and Wu (noon).
    - **Features**: Optimizes Qi flow by aligning it with specific times of the day, harmonizing the body's energy with natural cycles.
4. **Mao-You Jucheon (卯酉周天; Sunrise and Sunset Orbit)**:
    - **Pathway**: Practiced according to the time periods of Mao (dawn) and You (dusk).
    - **Features**: Circulates Qi during specific times, utilizing the energies of sunrise and sunset to optimize the body's energy.
5. **Dae Jucheon (大周天; Macrocosmic Orbit)**:
    - **Pathway**: Includes the Ren and Du Meridians of the Sojucheon and also involves circulating Qi through the twelve primary meridians throughout the body.

- **Features**: An advanced practice recommended after mastering the Sojucheon, enhancing Qi circulation throughout the entire body, leading to greater health and vitality.

6. Dan Do Jucheon (丹道周天; Dan Orbit):
    - **Pathway**: Focuses on alchemical transformations within the body, utilizing internal Qi and essence (Jeong) to cultivate spiritual and physical health.
    - **Features**: Emphasizes the integration of mind, body, and spirit, often involving complex visualizations and meditative techniques.

7. Geongon Jucheon (乾坤周天; Earth and Heaven Orbit):
    - **Pathway**: Symbolizes the interaction of Heaven (乾, ☰, GV 20) and Earth (坤, ☷, KD1), circulating Qi between these two fundamental forces.
    - **Features**: Aims to harmonize the practitioner's energy with the universal forces of Heaven and Earth, promoting a deep sense of unity with the cosmos. This practice can enhance spiritual insight and physical vitality.

These various Jucheon (Qi circulation orbit) practices offer a range of techniques for practitioners to explore, depending on their goals and level of experience.

Part III. Qigong Practice Journals & Testimonials

Irene Rizzini

Professor at Pontifical Catholic University of Rio de Janeiro
San Diego - Seminar at Idyllwild, Sep 2023

The next few pages summarize my experience during the seminar and a few days earlier, as I arrived in San Diego.

It is a challenge to express all that I experienced and felt in words. It was an intense experience—all concentrated in just a few days. But I will do my best.

I arrived in San Diego three days before the beginning of the seminar (August 29). That was good because I had some time to be close to Master Han and Jane after such a long time. They had been in Brazil in April 2017, and since then we have only been interacting via Zoom on Saturdays to practice Qigong. And I am grateful for that, because this way we were able to maintain a stronger sense of connection.

But to meet in person is completely different.

I especially miss the in-person learning and the possibility of energy exchange that happens when physically close and touched by the Master; that changes it all.

As I arrived, it was great to hug Jane as she picked me up. She took me directly to the studio where Master Han was teaching, and, to my surprise, I confess, they put me to practice right away. I was tired and a bit worried about meeting everyone and starting like that—like I was not really prepared. But Master Han immediately made me feel like I was part of the group, and all the students welcomed me warmly.

Even so, I was tense. After all these years and most of the time practicing on my own, what would Master Han think of my Tai Chi? I worried. It also feels different now that I am 69. I feel my body is very flexible and strong, but the reality is that we get older, and that affects us in different ways. Would I be able to enjoy the seminar even so? I was a bit insecure.

As I started, the first movements with the sword were awkward. Nothing seemed to flow well. I was nervous; the shoes were a bit large, and I found it hard to balance myself. But I kept going, as Master Han always tells us to do.

During these days, we had a gift from the full moon and a special one: the blue moon. I had never seen or felt it. Some of us went with Master Han and Jane for meditation in the open air—right in front of that round, big, and extremely bright moon. Meditating together felt good. The energy irradiated was amazing.

Maria, one of the students, came with us for meditation and for a meal. To meet her was a beautiful surprise, for we had such a brief interaction, but we both felt an incredible connection. She asked me what kind of work I did, and I saw that she was particularly interested. We started talking from there and discovered several points that connected us. We were both taken with emotion by this beautiful bond that quickly formed between us.

Besides Tai Chi, Master Han has introduced us to various forms of meditation and Qigong practices. I have been lucky to learn some over the years, and it all felt familiar to me. I first met Master Han in 2006, when I came to the US as a visiting scholar at the University of Notre Dame and spent time in Chicago. The way we met was an amazing story, but this is another story. But because it felt amazing to me and I felt close right away to Master Han, it made all the difference. He has been an important person in my life.

Seminar (September 1 to 4)

I will now summarize some experiences that I registered in my diary during the hours of intense practice at the seminar, combining hours of meditation (standing and sitting), Qigong, and Tai Chi (Lao jia).

Day 1 – Friday (1 September 2023)

We arrived at the place we were going to stay in mid-afternoon. Meeting the group felt good. And it was especially great to meet Brian after so many years and be able to talk and practice together. A diverse group, different generations, but all super committed and open to learning.

Master Han introduced us to practicing this same day during the evening.

First standing meditation (Mugeugjang) (for one hour)

I chose a place facing the garden and trees, and I think that helped me. I had walked by the river in the garden earlier and felt connected to the place. During the practice, I connected to the river through my roots. It was the first time that I saw my roots this clearly. They came down from my feet strongly—a purple and pinkish color, so natural in contact with the earth, leaves, other roots, and nature elements. It felt so good. My roots went down all the way to the river and further down. It was a cool sensation of freshness and dampness.

Standing for a long time was surprisingly easier for me this time. At first, I felt a bit like in the past, with my ankles and feet not really firm, particularly on the right side. But as Master Han approached, particularly when he pressed my shoulders and back down, I felt deeply grounded through my yongchun(Kd1; the ball of the foot). It was the first time I really felt so deeply grounded and stable.

After some time, I also felt enormous pressure on my spine (middle back), close to the heart and lungs. It was even a bit hard to breathe, as if I needed more air.

This sensation did not come back the other days while standing; in fact, I felt better each day.

The problem was more during the sitting meditations. I do not meditate in a sitting position regularly (in part because I sit many hours a day for work, writing, or reading). So, I prefer standing practices (Qigong, meditation, and Tai Chi). The pain in my back increased after the second day every time I sat for meditation. Fortunately, I had no pain at all while standing meditation and while practicing Tai Chi. Master Han helped me by pressing some points and with massage. That gave me immediate relief, and I could feel several knots on my back as he massaged it.

I told Master Han that I have been diagnosed as having hypothyroidism and that my doctor has been signaling that it has increased. I want to try to balance myself and not take stronger medication (what I take now is a very low dose). Master Han has pressed some points below my throat, and they did hurt a lot. But I am confident I will be able to improve with the current practices I have been learning.

Day 2 – Saturday (2 September 2023)

Sunrise meditation

It was easier than the first day, and it felt so good all over, both externally and internally. I chose a place in the form of a tree on the verandah, with the river below. My root connection was immediate and strong, directly to the river. This time I felt my heart beating, the blood pulsing, and a nice warmth in the palms of my hands.

Several 'images' popped into my mind during this practice. I think they were related to the meditation Master Han taught us, in which we are asked to reflect upon 'Who we really are'. All I know is that what came to me was good, and I do not know how to put it into words, but it all made sense to me. I simply know it.

I still felt more pressure on my right ankle and foot (as always), but a lot less. I wonder if this discomfort there, as well as on my back and right shoulder, is related to blockages that make the Qi find it hard to flow.

This morning, we went together uphill on a trail. It was so beautiful and complemented all we were practicing and learning. I went up and down just behind Jane and was able to hear the soothing music she was listening to. That gave the walk a special touch.

To dive into an intense experience like this, one has to be open and humble, for it is challenging and can also be frustrating. It is like we have to unlearn certain things to be able to learn others—this level of openness. This was most true when practicing Lao Jia (Chen Tai Chi Form). And this is because I practiced with different masters and groups in the past and got my own way of moving, frequently incorrectly, not really connected to my Dantian. So, to try to 'forget' how one normally moves and be open to letting the whole-body flow differently is wonderful, but not always possible. But this time, I understood it all better.

We had all our meals together. Easy conversation and sharing during these moments made us all feel closer, adding a nice group energy to our daily practices.

Day 3 - Sunday (3 September 2023)

Today I felt much more confident during the Tai Chi practice. Everything is flowing better. My Qi flowed more smoothly and strongly. I believe it is the impact of all the practices Master Han has been integrating (including more subtle inner practices) that produces an effect of wholeness, of embracing us fully (body, mind, soul, and spirit). The heart Qigong and the stomach Qigong added a lot more to my ongoing practice.

During the day, and particularly during the night sitting meditation, I felt a more acute pain in my back (middle). Master Han said something about being somehow related to my heart. I suspect this is true, but I really do not know. I believe, from what I have been learning, that a more fluid flow of the Qi will help me with all this in the long run.

This morning, we meditated in the lower area, by the river. I chose a spot at the top of a rock where the sun was shining brightly. It felt incredibly good.

And later, as we practiced standing poll meditation again, for the first time I saw and felt this bright spot of light in my lower Dantian.

Day 3 - Monday (4 September 2023)

Our last day.

It is time to say goodbye. At this point, the group was beautifully bonded. I still had some time in San Diego with Master Han and Jane, and I enjoyed every minute of it. And I ask you two to accept my deepest gratitude, not only for all this but also for being a very important part of my life!

Lisa Colette Martin

Artist and Interior Designer

I think it is somewhat universal that injury can take us on a journey. I had been suffering from degenerative spine disease pain since 2011, which increased at a rapid rate with each passing year. I opted to avoid surgery to 'fix' me because my spine specialist told me that I would find relief only in one area and only for a couple years before I would likely have to face it all over again. So, I made use of the normal western medicine remedies, mostly prescription pain relief drugs, specialist visits 2-3 times a year, acupuncture, and physical therapy. These were aimed at slowing the disease progression since I was told there was no cure for all the problems, I had that fell under the umbrella term 'degenerative spine disease.' In 2015, my pain level had become so bad that I could not stand up straight, could not lift my head off the ground when laying down, and I lost sleep nightly. I was in tears often, not able to hold back in front of friends. In 2015, I had the fortune of having a dear friend refer me to Master Sang Pok Han to help relieve pain. I didn't understand how Tai Chi could help, but I trusted my friend's sincerity and agreed to try it. Master Han took great interest in my well-being, as he does for all his students. With care not to further my injuries, he began to teach me how to 'get in touch' with the natural physiology of my body to begin a healing process through building strength gently, movement, and circulating energy. I had to have an open mind; little by little, each week, I was becoming stronger. Within six months, I was standing up straight again, losing the hunched-over stance that had become my norm. I was learning to slow down my mind and get in touch with my body and its natural inner workings. I paid more attention to how everything I think, do, and eat is connected to my health. The Golden Rishi group became a new family to me. What we shared was a pursuit of health, well-being, and authentic care for each other. I added the practice of Master Han's Qigong class to my life in 2017.

Tai Chi and Qigong complement each other; together and separately, the two disciplines foster a deeper understanding of our body. The understanding that I had gained through Master Han's coursework set the stage for receiving a miracle healing in 2018. The healing session was facilitated by Master Han's mentor, Grand Master Byung Joo Choi, in South Korea. I returned from that trip pain-free. As of the publishing date of this book, I am still pain-free, and I am and will always be part of the Golden Rishi family.

Austin W. Gunter

Technical Product Marketing Consultant

Doing Qigong and Tai Chi with Master Han has really transformed my life in a very short period of time. The more time I invest in meditation and learning the forms, the more energy I have, the happier I am, and the better the rest of my life is. I've been sensitive to "energy" for many years, and I can tell that both the modalities that Master Han teaches, as well as how much of a master he himself is connected to, are offering something powerful to my life.

Specifically, I have inflammation in my joints from an auto-immune disorder, and Master Han will come up to me during class and press on various acupressure points. It hurts a bit when he does this (sort of like a massage), but I can tell that he's activating something in my body and perhaps even offering some new energy to me. He does this a lot when we're practicing in the park, when we're getting all this good energy from the trees and nature.

I've had three different Tai Chi teachers over the past 10 years or so, and I can confidently say that Master Han is the best. I feel like we are very lucky to have him in San Diego, and I would suspect there are very few people in the world who have as much to teach and who love teaching as much as he does.

S. Vedder

M. A. in Education

I decided to search for a Qigong school at a time in my life when I realized that, because of my age and condition, if I didn't do something soon, I would not be able to enjoy a good level of health. For years, at every checkup with my physician, I'd been asked how often I exercised, and I wouldn't have much to say. My health had also been impacted by years of stress from work and of being too 'busy' to pay attention to my own fitness. Then, my stress and fitness became more negatively impacted when I was faced with several losses in my life.

And so I finally looked for something to do that would help me. I remembered a demonstration of Qigong I had seen once that had impressed me, so I checked for a local class. I tried a sample Golden Rishi class, and it was enough to convince me to enroll. As I first started classes, my main goal was to relieve stress. When I went to class, I would simply follow without thinking, and focus on breathing and motions. I felt like I was in a different realm. Meditation always made me feel better, even if I couldn't understand why. After a while, as soon as I entered the dojo, I could feel my shoulders relax, and I would naturally breathe deeper.

After relieving stress, I realized I needed to work on balance and flexibility. My body, after years of caregiving, was weak and I had lost some mobility which was quite upsetting. In class, I was encouraged to do as much as I was able to try a little harder, and gradually but steadily I improved. Because of the relaxed and welcoming atmosphere in class, I felt comfortable to start at my level, build on it, and keep on going. This helped me to persevere and become stronger.

My stamina and strength are now much better, in some cases like that of my younger self, and in some ways maybe even better (though in others I still have a long way to go). I have dealt with broken bones, shoulder tears, knee issues, etc., and have found Qigong to take the place of many Western medical approaches. It is also enlightening and hopeful. It doesn't tell me that my health issues are just part of growing older. It helps me understand how everything in the body is connected or related, and what I can do to help my body do its work of healing itself.

Tai Chi has been a part of my journey. Practicing Tai Chi while practicing Qigong has enhanced my understanding and ability. I have figured out that practice is its own reward. It has taken lots of practice for me to learn the beginning levels, but that is the point–to keep practicing. At one point I started taking notes and writing reflections after class to accelerate my progress. Other students offered their tips, and have encouraged me greatly, too. But the point is not to get somewhere but to keep the practice up for its own recurring benefits.

Now, not only do I feel more fit and invigorated, but my standard health indicators show impressive changes. My cholesterol was lowered 50 points, blood pressure is now at a good level, no more broken bones, heart palpitations gone, sleep improved. I never expected that this much improvement could be realized!

I am so grateful that I found this wonderful Golden Rishi Qigong program. Master Han and the Golden Rishi team are exemplary. Master Han shares the proficiency he gained in years of study. His teaching and leadership styles are of outstanding quality. He is responsible, caring, kind, encouraging, and he adjusts high standards for each student. The instruction guides students in a step-by-step manner and is based on centuries of learning. Additionally, at Golden Rishi, there is personal attention, choice, and a family atmosphere, which creates a cohort of learners who are unique individuals, all trying to improve themselves, build on commonalities, and be of benefit to others.

Many blessings.

(For fun) –My Life Lessons from Tai Chi & Qigong

1. Set intention first.
2. Keep a level head.
3. Place your feet solidly so that you can be stable and stand firm.
4. Leaning is weakness. (Keep your spine straight.)
5. All movements and actions must be based in or anchored to the core (dantian).
6. Don't react to an attack with an opposite action; try instead to deflect it or get it off balance.
7. Keep loose knees and shoulders.
8. All movements are linked with other parts of the body.
9. Focus on getting the big movements and refine later.
10. Practice and it will come.
11. Force comes from the core being the base of other movements.
12. Energy moves in spiral patterns to stay strong and not dissipate.
13. Lead with the dantian.
14. Arms defend the core and return to center between movements.
15. Walk like a ninja: solid feet/steps, quiet, strong, low ('sink').

16. Set pace based on breathing.
17. Place one foot firmly, transfer weight, then move the other foot.
18. Practice.
19. Always spine straight.
20. Keep your body strong, as if defending it from a push or pull.
21. Make legs and arms strong to assist the heart.
22. Strength is inside softness.
23. We are born with energy, then it becomes blocked within us.
24. Qigong balances the body, builds muscle, has a self-healing and a meditative effect which trains us to better see inside the body–it sets our energy free.

Arsh Chopra, M.D.

Cardiothoracic Anesthesiologist

As a student of Master Han, I have been fortunate to learn from him directly. The publication of Qigong extends this opportunity to a broader audience. Over the course of the book, Master Han shepherds' readers through a transformative wellness journey. Consistent with his customary teachings, his writing provides an in-depth foundation of the history and roots of Qigong practice.

Readers of this book may have pursued improved wellness by other routes and methods. Unique to Qigong is a comprehensive approach that adds dimension by interlacing spirituality with anatomy and physiology as a determinant of health. In doing so, Master Han explores an approach to health, humanity and being that is underrepresented in Western society. Though suitable for individuals from all backgrounds, audiences will find that Qigong offers a new frontier on wellness – one that complements more popularized strategies.

As denoted in the title, with steady practice, one's vital energy can be cultivated through the teachings of Master Han. It is my pleasure to recommend this work, and my hope that doing so assists countless individuals to benefit as I have.

David Bach, M.D.

Neuroscientist and Founder and President of Optios

During my life, I've had the opportunity to study with several extraordinary teachers in a broad array of arenas. Based on that experience, I feel confident in saying that Master Han is one of the most special teachers with whom I've ever had the privilege of working.

I first discovered Tai Chi and Qigong in 2010, when I was living in New York City. From the moment that I took my first Tai Chi class, I felt a powerful "resonance" with the practice that I simply can't explain, and that no other physical practice has ever been able to touch. For a few years after I took my first Tai Chi class, I found myself diving into the practice quite deeply, even getting to the point where I was able to compete (e.g., in push hands) in a few local competitions.

Unfortunately, due to a confluence of life-events, including a decision to start a new company as well as a move to San Diego, I stopped doing Tai Chi in 2014 ... but in the back of my mind, even as I was doing lots of other physical practices (like yoga), I always knew I wanted to go back to Tai Chi and Qigong at some point.

I took my first class at Golden Rishi in early 2023, and from the moment I walked in the door there, I knew I had found a new "home."

In addition to the fact that Master Han is, clearly, the "real deal" (his depth of knowledge is almost staggering), what I particularly love about the Golden Rishi studio is the "energy" in their classes. It is not a stretch to say that Master Han and Jane are almost pure beings of light. And on top of that, their students – who, of course, also make up an important part of the experience – are serious in their practice, while also immensely welcoming to newcomers, which, in my experience, is a rare combination.

As of this writing, I have been studying at Golden Rishi for a little over a year now, and I also practice regularly at home. I feel immensely grateful to have the opportunity to work with Master Han and Jane, and on top of that, it is almost staggering how much better and happier my body, mind and spirit all feel as a direct result of these practices.

Maria Tong

Tai Chi and Qigong Instructor

When Chen Style Tai Chi and Qigong entered into my life, I had limited knowledge of this thousand-year-old eastern practice. It began as a desire to spend quality time with my family, since it was difficult to balance home, a demanding job as an international flight attendant, and raising sons with my husband. I thought Tai Chi looked simple, but soon, I realized Tai Chi offered benefits beyond physical exercise. It is an internal martial art that emphasizes martial efficacy and Chinese philosophy.

Unfortunately, a couple of years later, I was struck by a brain hemorrhage, and my life changed overnight. I had numerous appointments with various doctors. Progress was slow and difficult. About one and a half years later, with low energy, limited motion, countless headaches, stomach issues, numbness and tingling in my hands and feet, I returned to Tai Chi. Master Han took all my ailments into consideration and we slowly began with modified movements to my ability. He was gentle, and very patient. I could only do 20-minute increments in the beginning, but as the time went on, I was gaining focus, balance, and strength.

A couple of years later, Master Han's Qigong teacher and healer Grandmaster Choi came from Korea and conducted a Qigong seminar. I was eager to meet and study Qigong, knowing he could assist in my healing. The seminar was conducted indoors and outdoors, using nature's energy to help ourselves to cultivate our own energy(qi).

Thanks to the previous Tai Chi training, my body and mind were ready to receive what I needed for the Qigong seminar. I was able to follow and begin to really feel the effects of meditation. For the first time ever, I could sit for forty-five minutes straight, and not have a monkey mind. As the days went on, meditations were more intensive but easier. On the last night of meditation, I had a breakthrough. I knew that from that moment on, I could aid in the healing process by myself, if I continued on this path of learning Tai Chi and Qigong. I was presented with a certificate for completing the Golden Rishi Qigong for achieving the level as the first North American women. I was overjoyed with happy tears. When we returned home, I went to my chiropractor neurology doctor. As soon as my doctor saw me, his eyes widened with a surprised look. He said, "What have you done? You are glowing and you look like you have less pain. Whatever you are doing, keep doing it." His comments confirmed that my progress was due to Tai Chi and Qi Gong since he had no idea that I had gone to a Qigong seminar.

The knowledge I have gained through eastern methods of self-healing with western medicine, has left me with a realization that, no matter what we struggle with in life, if one is willing and open minded, we can find our own healing modality with guidance from wonderful teachers like Master Han and Grandmaster Choi. Therefore, I highly recommend Tai Chi and Qigong to anyone who is interested.

Jinhee Muren

Artist & Tai Chi Instructor of Southwestern College

My most valuable lesson from Master Han is his example of limitless patience and empathy with and for others. This is regardless of each student's background, situation in life and physical ability. He consistently maintains a positive relationship with his students.

I was not a patient person when I began to learn Tai Chi with Master Han ten years ago. Instead of practicing to refine the same movements, forms and techniques that had I just learned, I would ask what the next step is. I was wrongly focusing on just advancing through a routine instead of striving for the benefits that come with intentional practice. I also had doubts. I did not believe Tai Chi and Qigong practice could increase the energy level in our human body. Through my beginning attempts, nothing made sense to me, so practicing Tai Chi challenged me in every aspect of my life.

Learning Tai Chi was an unexpected opportunity through friends. It took me a long time to realize the program offers an intricate design of balance for healthy human existence. It is not only to build up physical strength but building up mental faculties as well. Emotional and physical journey through each person's life includes suffering and joy; for me I've come to believe through the Golden Rishi coursework that sometimes we must lose something to experience gain. That is part of life, just like the extremes of light versus dark. Eventually, I learned that Tai Chi is the one of the best modalities to reach discipline in health, and in life. Tai Chi leans on martial arts in a way that we meditate while in motion. The meditation process is one in which the universal energy that exists in constant rotation all around us naturally circulates. As I came to understand the powerful methods of Tai Chi and Qigong, my discipline and strength developed.

I have learned so much from Master Han about mindset, patience, and ultimate health that I am now teaching Tai Chi at a community college now. I wish to share what I have learned with others, and this is a way to do so. The opportunity and drive to teach is another unexpected life changing experience that came from my association with Master Han. I have many students with disabilities and limited mobility. Watching Master Han's students and teaching Tai Chi myself, I have realized there are no restrictions on age, strength level, or [dis]ability when learning Tai Chi. Movements, deep breathing, and relaxation techniques can be modified to slow routines and increase awareness of a student's surroundings. I am a witness that Tai Chi and Qigong can help anyone's life.

I find this journey to be enjoyable and invigorating. Master Han encourages and compels me to continue learning and to refine my technique and skill set. I know this will lead me to achieve higher levels of mastery over time.

Heesoo Kim

Ph.D. in Linguistics

I have been learning Qi Gong and Tai Chi from Master Han. Until you get a haircut, you don't really feel how much your hairs weigh. When you enter a warm room and relax on a winter day, you finally realize how tiring it is to shiver with cold outside was. Just like these, practicing Tai Chi and Qi Gong with Master Han, I am learning how to relax, realizing how much tension I have been carrying in my body all my life. My hands were cold throughout the year, but now, 5 min after I started Dantian breathing, my hands start warming up. They stay warm throughout the night if I do Dantian breathing right before going to bed. During the day, my hands still tend to be cold, which is why I need to keep practicing relaxation through Dantian breathing. Qi Gong focuses on restoring your intrinsic balance and circulation with your body and mind relaxed, while Tai Chi teaches you how to relax under physical challenges. This is why Qi Gong is best for healing and Tai Chi is great for making you stronger if you are already relatively healthy. If you do both Qi Gong and Tai Chi hand in hand, it is ideal of course. You just have no idea what a huge blessing it truly is to be able to learn from Master Han, a man of the highest integrity I've ever seen. Training with him can be literally life-changing!

Larry Tong

Tai Chi and Qigong Instructor

I once met an old sage, and I asked him "What is Qigong?" He said, "Imagine a big bowl of sand. Each grain represents some cure, remedy, medicine, diet, or exercise routine. Along came a great wind and it blew all the sand out. The only thing left standing was the bowl." I quickly interjected, "Was Qigong in the bowl and it was scattered with the wind?" The wise sage just smiled and responded, "No, the bowl is Qigong."

The story relates that Qigong is all encompassing. It has been around for thousands of years. The basis for all the cures, diets and exercises are based on Qigong principles of rebalancing oneself back to universal nature.

If you have done any research on Qigong, you probably found that there is a lot of information on the subject. These books, videos and teaching guides are an important part of the legacy of Qigong that is passed to each new generation. It is important to acknowledge the people that have strived to keep the benefits of Qigong available to those who had the desire to learn.

During my lifetime, I was fortunate enough to meet the founders of Golden Rishi. Grand master Choi and Master Han are vital contributors to the preservation of the history, study, and practice of Qigong. They have spent countless hours studying to improve and distill the most important facets of the art. Golden Rishi Qigong is now shared and practiced at an international level. Dedicated students continue to pass it on to the next generations.

Qigong for me has been like a new journey. When you plan to visit a new city, you read the guidebooks that describe the highlights of the city. When you get there, you can schedule a bus tour, or you can drive yourself to all the main attractions. But I found that if you really want to get to know a city and its people, you must get out and walk. Qigong is similar as you can read books and watch movies about its benefits but to truly understand Qigong you must experience it. While you are walking around the new city you are visiting you are experiencing the daily life of the people who live there. Now, how much more would you be able to learn and experience with a qualified tour guide? Qigong is the same, you can try to practice on your own through trial and error or you can find a suitable teacher who can guide you through the experience. I had an interest in Qigong from when I was young, I read books I could find on the subject. It was a good background, but it really started to fall into place once I started practicing with Golden Rishi.

It is hard to describe the exhilaration when you initially start to become aware of this pulsating energy sensation. I noticed it quite strongly at Presidio Park where we were doing the first Qigong seminar. I had to ask myself if it was real. It wasn't something I could see at the time, but I could feel as if I was pushing something invisible and it was pushing back! When I continued to practice, I noticed that depending on what you were doing the feeling was stronger than at other times. Over time, with continued practice and becoming more aware of the surroundings the feelings became more consistent. As time went on, explanations of what seemed to be complicated subject matter became more like common sense. It was as if you were now thinking with a Qigong brain.

My experience with Qigong has been nothing short of amazing. I had started training in Tai Chi several years prior to starting Qigong. The two arts complement each other so well. I always believed that Tai Chi set up the basis for me to transition to Qigong. Tai Chi is my Yang and Qigong my Yin. I will be forever indebted to Grand Master Choi and Master Han for taking their time to show me the best of each. I can only describe them as two living treasures that I had the fortune to meet.

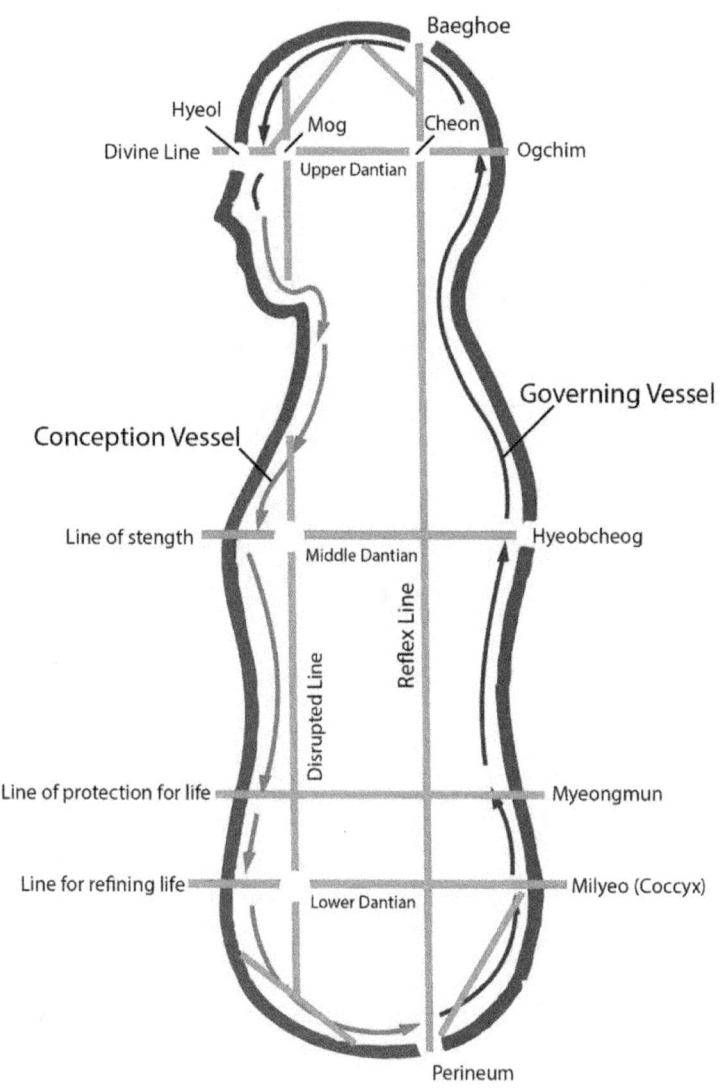

Inner Energy Chart